Keto Diet After 50

Keto for Seniors

*The Complete Guide to Burn Fat, Lose Weight,
and Prevent Diseases - With Simple 30 Minute
Keto Recipes and a 30-Day Meal Plan*

Table Of Contents

Introduction

Face it – we all struggled with weight problems at some point in our life. In fact, some people still struggle with weight loss and would happily lose a few more pounds, if given the chance. I definitely did. As I found out, the ability to lose the excess fat became more difficult as I got older. Metabolism slows down and physical activity starts to decrease so all those calories stack up and lodge themselves everywhere – belly, thighs, arms, neck, chin, and so on. Even if I wanted to exercise and lose all those excess fat – it isn't really possible because, well, exercise makes me feel constant chronic pain. I try to take a relaxing 3 minute walk and feel my legs and thighs throbbing for the rest of the day.

So what did I do? I did my research and found out that adopting a good diet for weight loss is usually the best solution. In fact, studies show that what you eat is more important than exercise when it comes to maintaining a healthy weight. The question here is – what kind of diet should I follow if I'm approaching my later years?

I tried winging it first – not following a specific diet but just making consciously healthy decisions. When that didn't work, I tried several diet types like the Paleo Diet, the Vegetarian route, and I even tried going Vegan. Finally, I decided to go to my doctor (which I should have done in the first place) and he told me to try the Ketogenic Diet, given my diabetic background. Since this was recommended by my doctor, I decided to be a wee bit more dedicated to the diet – and I started losing the excess weight! Before starting the Ketogenic Diet, I weighed 220 pounds, which for my height of 6 feet, puts me in the overweight category. In fact, if I went one pound over, I'd be obese.

Now, I'm at a healthy 190 pounds, and all credit goes to the Ketogenic Diet lifestyle. I want to share this discovery with everyone by introducing this new diet dubbed as the Ketogenic Diet.

It's not exactly brand new – but it is definitely one of the most effective methods of losing weight and gaining better health nowadays. Since I started the Ketogenic Diet, I managed to lose 30 pounds, have better clarity, experience less foggy days, and even wake up in the morning feeling completely refreshed. If you're like me – then chances are you've woken up in the morning and you feel just as tired as you did the night before.

I want you to know that this is not a fly by night creation. I personally went through this and it is NOT easy. However, the results are so wonderfully satisfying that I felt it my duty to share this information with the world.

Don't believe me? Do your research the same way I did. Many medical publications today talk about the advantages of going on the Ketogenic Diet. These studies consider many factors related to the dietary plan such as how it compares with a low-carbohydrate approach or a low-calorie approach.

In this book, I've made every effort to communicate what I know and have learned after years of enjoying the benefits of the Ketogenic Diet. If you've read Keto books before and became frustrated about the in-depth and complicated explanations – don't worry anymore! I've made sure that this book is as simple and as straightforward, giving you only what is considered essential in order to make the most out of the Ketogenic Diet.

But that's enough talking – read on and find out exactly what you can enjoy even as you enter your older years!

Chapter 1: How the Ketogenic Diet Works

What Is the Ketogenic Diet?

The Ketogenic Diet actually follows a fairly simple principle: keep your food consumption low-carb and high-fat. So basically, being on the diet means eating less carbohydrates and adding more fats in your daily meals. Don't be confused. When we say "fat" we're not talking about the literal kind that's attached to your body. Fat has gotten a bad reputation nowadays, but "fat" the nutrient is actually very different from the "fat" that makes your clothes fit tight.

Good fats are the kind you get from avocado, nuts, and fish. For example, there are the omega-3 and omega-6 fatty acids that actually help you lose weight, get better heart health, and have excellent hair and nails.

What Happens to Your Body When You Eat Keto?

Even before we talk about how to do keto – it's important to first consider why this particular diet works. What actually happens to your body to make you lose weight?

As you probably know, the body uses food as an energy source. Everything you eat is turned into energy, so that you can get up and do whatever you need to accomplish for the day. The main energy source is sugar so what happens is that you eat something, the body breaks it down into sugar, and the sugar is processed into energy. Typically, the "sugar" is taken directly from the food you eat so if you eat just the right amount of food, then your body is fueled for the whole day. If you eat too much, then the sugar is stored in your body – hence the accumulation of fat.

But what happens if you eat less food? This is where the Ketogenic Diet comes in. You see, the process of creating sugar from food is usually faster if the food happens to be rich in carbohydrates. Bread, rice, grain, pasta – all of these are carbohydrates and they're the easiest food types to turn into energy.

So the Ketogenic Diet is all about reducing the amount of carbohydrates you eat. Does this mean you won't get the kind of energy you need for the day? Of course not! It only means that now, your body has to find other possible sources of energy. Do you know where they will be getting that energy? Your stored body fat!

So here's the situation – you are eating less carbohydrates every day. To keep you energetic, the body breaks down the stored fat and turns them into molecules called ketone bodies. The process of turning the fat into ketone bodies is called "Ketosis" and obviously – this is where the name of the Ketogenic Diet comes from. The ketone bodies take the place of glucose in keeping you energetic. As long as you keep your carbohydrates reduced, the body will keep getting its energy from your body fat.

Sounds Simple, Right?

The Ketogenic Diet is often praised for its simplicity and when you look at it properly, the process is really straightforward. The Science behind the effectivity of the diet is also well-documented, and has been proven multiple times by different medical fields. For example, an article on Diet Review by Harvard provided a lengthy discussion on how the Ketogenic Diet works and why it is so effective for those who choose to use this diet.

But Fat Is the Enemy...Or Is It?

No – fat is NOT the enemy. Unfortunately, years of bad science told us that fat is something you have to avoid – but it's actually a very helpful thing for weight loss! Even before we move forward with this book, we'll have to discuss exactly what "healthy fats" are, and why they're actually the good guys. To do this, we need to make a distinction between the different kinds of fat. You've probably heard of them before and it is a little bit confusing at first. We'll try to go through them as simply as possible:

Saturated fat. This is the kind you want to avoid. They're also called "solid fat" because each molecule is packed with hydrogen atoms. Simply put, it's the kind of fat that can easily cause a blockage in your body. It can raise cholesterol levels and lead to heart problems or a stroke. Saturated fat is something you can find in meat, dairy products, and other processed food items. Now, you're probably wondering: isn't the Ketogenic Diet packed with saturated fat? The answer is: not necessarily. You'll find later in the recipes given that the Ketogenic Diet promotes primarily unsaturated fat or healthy fat. While there are definitely many meat recipes in the list, most of these recipes contain healthy fat sources.

Unsaturated Fat. These are the ones dubbed as healthy fat. They're the kind of fat you find in avocado, nuts, and other ingredients you usually find in Keto-friendly recipes. They're known to lower blood cholesterol and actually come in two types: polyunsaturated and monounsaturated. Both are good for your body but the benefits slightly vary, depending on what you're consuming.

Polyunsaturated fat. These are perhaps the best in the list. You know about omega-3 fatty acids right? They're often suggested for people who have heart problems and are recognized as the "healthy" kind of fat. Well, they fall under the category of polyunsaturated fat and are known for reducing risks of heart disease by as much as 19 percent. This is according to a study titled: Effects on coronary heart diseases of increased poly-unsaturated fat in lieu of saturated fat: systematic review & meta-analysis of randomized controlled tests. So where do you get these polyunsaturated fats? You can get them mostly from vegetable and seed oils. These are ingredients you can almost always find in Ketogenic Recipes such as olive oil, coconut oil, and more. If you need more convincing, you should also know that omega-3 fatty acids are actually a kind of polyunsaturated fats and you will find them in deep sea fish like tuna, herring, and salmon.

Chapter 2: Benefits of Going on a Ketogenic Diet

So what exactly can you look forward to once you go on a Ketogenic Diet? There are tons of benefits! Here are some of the pros of this brand new diet:

Efficient Way to Lose Weight

Let's forget calories for a few minutes and just concentrate on the kind of nutrients you have in your food. A study published in PubMed which allows for a *meta-analysis of randomized controlled trial between a very-low carbohydrate ketogenic diet versus a low-fat diet for long term weight loss* shows that the low-carb option provides for better long-term results. It can even help reduce risk factors of cardiovascular problems, which simply means that you'll have less chances of suffering from heart problems or high blood pressure.

The science behind this isn't that complicated. The fact is that the body finds it easier to turn sugar into energy – which is why when given the choice, your body will always choose to run on sugar. Fat is also a possible source of energy – but it takes more work, which is why you lose weight more consistently with a Ketogenic Diet.

Reduces the Risk of Acne

You'd think a person in their 50's wouldn't have acne – and you'd probably be right. Note though that a large part of what you eat affects skin health, even if you're already in your 50s. In fact, people in their 50s need to be extra careful with skin health because this is when growths, blackheads, pore blockages, and more become persistent. Studies show that rapid changes in blood sugar have an effect on skin health as discussed in a study titled: *Nutrition and acne – therapeutic potential of ketogenic diets.*

May Help Reduce Cancer Risks

Switching to the Ketogenic Diet may help reduce the risk of cancer, especially as the risk of it increases upon reaching the age of 50. Although that's just a small percentage, it's definitely worth noting – especially if you happen to have a history of cancer in the family. It's also interesting to note that the Ketogenic Diet is usually prescribed as a complement to chemotherapy. A study titled *"Ketogenic diets as an adjuvant cancer therapy: history and potential mechanism"* concluded that the deprivation of sugar causes more stress to the cancer cells. This simply means that cancer cells depend more on the glucose you have on your body and once their energy source is cut-off, they're more likely to die off.

Reduces Risk of Heart Problems

Healthy fat found in avocado, nuts, and other food items promoted by the Ketogenic Diet can help reduce the possibility of heart problems. In a study titled: The long-term effects of a ketogenic diet in obese patients, it was seen that going on a Keto Diet significantly increases HDL and lowers LDL. HDL is known as the "good cholesterol" while LDL is the "bad cholesterol" known for increasing the likelihood of heart problems. So does this mean that all fat is healthy? No. Remember, we're only talking about the good fat here as previously discussed. The bad type are still discouraged and are not part of the Ketogenic Diet.

Protects Brain Function

Have you ever found yourself trying to remember simple things – like what things to buy from the store or what day to pay the power bill? Forgetfulness becomes more common as you grow older – but it doesn't have to be! In a study titled: The effects of Ketogenic Diet on behavior and cognition, it was revealed that children following the diet have better cognitive functioning and alertness. It's also theorized that the diet has neurological protective benefits – which basically means that it can help prevent problems that affect brain function. For example, you'll have slightly lower risks of Parkinson's, Alzheimer's, and other forms of dementia.

Bone Health

Osteoporosis becomes more likely as a person advances in age. This is especially true if you weren't able to introduce appropriate amounts of calcium in your body. As you probably known, osteoporosis makes the bone brittle and fragile. This means that your likelihood of having serious injury from seemingly small accidents increases. A simple slip and bones can fracture or hips may become dislocated. Persistent inflammation of the joints could become an everyday problem. The Ketogenic Diet is a good way of preventing these from happening because the diet naturally involves the intake of healthy dairy or milk products. More importantly, the Ketogenic Diet promotes the intake of low-toxin food products. Hence, your body absorbs food nutrients better, ensuring that all the minerals you need is distributed evenly throughout the body.

But I'm Over 50!

I understand that you have several concerns when using the Ketogenic Diet. Sure, the benefits are definitely great – but many of these benefits are experienced by those who are in their 40s or younger. This means that aside from the excess weight, they don't really have any other health problems to contend with. But what if you're already in your 50s or more? From what I see, most people in their 50s already have several health issues. Usually, these are health problems that occur simply because of age – so don't feel too bad about yourself!

For example, high blood pressure, heart problems, and diabetes are common problems for people in their 50s. If you happen to be this situation – it's important to first consult your doctor before going on the Ketogenic Diet – or any other diet for that matter. Since we're doing our best to cover all areas of Ketogenic Diet for people over 50, this book will also talk about some of the downsides if you have existing health problems. As someone who has done extensive research and have a ton of personal experiences from working with clients, I want you to know that there is absolutely NOTHING to be afraid of when switching to this brand new dietary plan.

Check out the next Chapter and find out what else to expect with this new diet!

Chapter 3: Ketogenic Diet for People Over 50

I've encountered instances where a person wants to go on a Ketogenic Diet but hesitated because they have pre-existing health problems. As mentioned, if you're in your 50s, you likely have several health problems and even if you don't, you still have to be extra careful with any new lifestyle choice. Even when exercising, older individuals have to choose workouts that don't put too much strain on the bones and muscles!

In this Chapter therefore, we're going to consider the use of Ketogenic Diet if you've been diagnosed with health problems or at a risk for it or if you're just 50 years old or above.

Keto for People with Diabetes

We've already mentioned this – Keto is good for people with diabetes. In fact, this is the primary reason why the Ketogenic Diet was recommended to me by my doctor. The science behind this is fairly straightforward – people with diabetes usually have high levels of sugar in their body. As mentioned, what food type is the quickest source of sugar for the body? Carbohydrates! Simply put, people with diabetes eat lots of carbohydrates, causing their blood sugar to rise and over time, it develops into diabetes. Note though, we're talking about Type 2 Diabetes here which occurs due to diet. Type 1 Diabetes has something to do with the hormones and is usually controlled through medication.

With the Ketogenic Diet, you're basically swapping the carbohydrates for a healthier and more sustainable option. This doesn't just sound good in theory though – there have been studies done on this and it was proven multiple times by the scientific community. In fact, you might find that some doctors recommend the Ketogenic Diet to the diabetic patients (like me). In a study published in Nutrition and Metabolism titled *"The effect of a low-carb diet, ketogenic diet vs. low-glycemic index diet on blood sugar control in Type 2 Diabetics"*, it was concluded that the Ketogenic Diet actually led to improvements on sugar control.

It's also important to note that diabetes is a problem that increases the risk of other health issues. Basically, this means that if you have diabetes, then there's a good chance that you'll also develop other health problems in the future – like high blood pressure and heart problems.

Note that even people with diabetes can have a low blood sugar. In fact, if you have diabetes and go on a Keto diet, there's a good chance that the blood sugar *will* dip to levels that are no longer healthy. Again, this is why we encourage diabetics to go to the doctor first before doing any kind of diet.

The Calorie and Nutrient Balance

Do you know why else the Ketogenic Diet is good for you specifically, as someone who just hit 50 years of age? What you should keep in mind is that as a person advances in age, their calorie needs decrease. For example, instead of 2,000 calories per day – you'll need only 1,800 calories per day. Why is that? Well, when we start to age –our physical activity significantly decreases. Hence, we don't need as much energy in our system. However, that doesn't mean our nutrient needs also go down. We still need the same amount of vitamins and minerals.

The Ketogenic Diet manages to hit a balance between these two needs. You get high nutrition for every calorie you get – which means that you'll maintain a decent amount of weight without really feeling less energetic for day to day activities.

Chapter 4: Ketogenic Diet FAQs

Why are you here?

OK – first things first – why are you here? I mean, why are you reading this book? Do you want to lose weight or do you want to just have a healthier lifestyle? This is an important question to ask and in all honesty, I feel like this is a question that we should have addressed in the first stage of the book.

If you'll notice, the book talks about how you can burn fat, lose weight, and prevent diseases with the Ketogenic Diet. Following this dietary plan will give you all three of these results – but finding out your ultimate goal will help you better plan your diet to achieve those goals. For example, if you're already happy with your weight and only want to have a healthier lifestyle, then you don't have to adhere so strictly to the carbohydrate requirement.

This is why I always encourage going to your primary physician first to find out what your dietary limits are. This was the first mistake I made when I decided to follow a weight loss regiment. Keep in mind – we're trying to improve the quality of your life and not make it worse.

Is there such a thing as too much fat?

Everything in moderation. If you consume too much of one thing, it doesn't matter even if its water – it will be too bad for you. So yes, you can eat too much fat – even if it's healthy fat as already discussed. Remember how we talked about the importance of calories? Well, you have to understand that of all the nutrients found today, fat is perhaps the most compact type. This means that each gram of fat has more calories than any other nutrients you can find today.

What does this mean? This means that if you eat too much fat, there's a good chance that you'll go beyond your calorie requirements. If your goal is weight loss or maintaining a healthy weight, then this is a bad route to take because you won't be experiencing a calorie deficit. Simply put – you'd actually gain weight instead of losing it. I want you to understand this because I don't want you eating more than you should in the mistaken belief that its "healthy" for you.

How much weight can you lose?

The amount of weight you can lose on the Ketogenic Diet depends primarily on how well you stick to the plan. The healthy rate is 2 pounds per week and I strongly recommend that you don't speed it up too much. As mentioned, I lost 30 pounds on the diet – but this took years of hard work and personal research on my part!

Should I be counting calories?

Generally, counting calories is the go-to for people who want to lose weight. You will find however that this is not a problem when you're on a Keto Diet. That doesn't mean you should forget calories altogether – it only means that it's not that big of an issue in the grand scheme of things.

So the question is – how many calories should you be eating if you're on a Ketogenic Diet? Well, this depends from one person to the next. You will find that there are calculators that can help you get the proper amount of calories you want to maintain while on Keto. A good online calculator is known as the Mifflin St. Jeor calculator which allows for a calorie suggestion based on your height, weight, and age.

Of course, if you want to be challenged, here's the typical formula.

For males: 10 multiplied by weight in kilograms + 6.25 x height in centimeters less 5 multiplied by age + 5

For females: 10 multiplied by weight in kilograms + 6.25 x height in centimeters less 5 multiplied by age – 161

Once you get the results, you'll have to multiply it using the following situations:

- Sedentary: x 1.2, if you have minimal physical activities such as having a desk job
- Lightly active: x 1.375 light jogging at least once a week
- Moderately active: x 1.55 moderate activity, at least 6 times a week
- Very active: x 1.725 hard exercise daily or hard exercise twice a week

So it's a little tough – but the online calculator should make the whole thing easier. Generally however, you'd want to maintain a calorie count of 1500 calories per day for weight loss. For health maintenance without the need to lose weight, you can hit 1800 to 2000 calories – depending on the level of activity you experience every day.

Here's the most important question however: do you have to be strict about it? The short answer is: YES. Just because you're on the Ketogenic Diet doesn't mean you can eat all the meat you want. This is not a free pass – you still have to be mindful of what you eat.

The good news is that if you follow the Ketogenic Diet strictly, you'll find that the period of satiation is longer. Simply put, you won't feel hungry so quickly on the diet. There will be no mid-afternoon cravings for a snack as you feel full all through the hours between lunch and dinner. Even if you *do* feel hungry, there are a bunch of Keto-friendly snacks you can reach for.

Chapter 5: Primary Keto Guidelines – the Do's and Don'ts of Keto Over 50

The Ketogenic Diet isn't as complicated as you would think. The general guidelines are simple and straightforward. Even for someone already in their 50s, the Keto Principle works just as well. Sure, there might be a need to make a few tweaks here and there to guarantee compatibility – but for the most part, everything one needs is easy to access.

What do we mean by that? Well, think about it – a person in their 50s is likely to have several maintenance medicines to help with their health. I know I've been taking several medications to help with problems like blood pressure, blood sugar, and so on. Once I made the decision to start a Ketogenic Diet, all of these medicines have to be taken into consideration. Like, is it OK to limit my food if I'm taking XXX medicine?

Of course, that's actually just one of the things I had to keep in mind. Here are other things you definitely have to consider when starting this brand new dietary lifestyle.

Do Consult Your Doctor Beforehand

I can't stress this enough – especially for people who fall into a certain age group. Your general practitioner will know your medical history better, your current health status, and whether going on a Ketogenic Diet would be a good idea. It's important to remember that any diet has an impact on things like your mental health and psychological health. The change from a regular carb-full diet to a carb-free one can create pressure on yourself, not just physically and mentally. Simply put, this means that if you're under any sort of stress – the dietary change can do more harm than good. Your general doctor would be able to consider all these factors and give good guidance. At the very least, they can make slight changes to the Ketogenic Diet Principles to meet your health needs.

Do Eat Less Than 50 Grams of Carbohydrates

The whole point of going on a Ketogenic Diet is to force the body to enter that state of Ketosis. To do that, one has to eat less than 50 grams of carbohydrates in a day. To put that in perspective, you should know that a single slice of white bread contains 49 grams of carbohydrates! Hence, people who are used to eating sandwiches for their meals are already eating way beyond the required limit. To let you better understand the low-carbohydrate principle, you should also note that the typical American eats around 225 to 325 grams of carbohydrates every day. For a healthy person with a normal weight, eating carbohydrates of around 225 to 325 is not a problem. For people trying to lose weight however, this amount should definitely be reduced.

Do Increase Your Fat Intake

When we say fat, we're talking about the healthy kind of fat. We already talked about this in a previous Chapter so I won't explain it so exhaustively this time. Try to stay away from products that are labeled as "fat free" because this is often packed with starchy ingredients.

Do Eat the Good Kind of Meat

Here's the good news for those following the Ketogenic Diet – meat is your friend. However, meat is you friendly only if it's the basic kind. What does this mean? Well, anything processed is not a good idea. You'd want to buy something that's as close to the real thing as possible. Sausages, hotdogs, and other meat products that went through a curing or preservation process are discouraged. If you can buy one directly from the farm, then that would be perfect.

Do Avoid Excessive Exercise

Especially during the first few weeks of keto, try not to exercise or do anything strenuous. I want you to focus on the diet to help yourself better stay faithful to the meal plan.

This is because if you push yourself to exercise AND follow the Ketogenic Diet, there's a good chance that you'll fail in both. Pour all your willpower into keeping with the meal plans, even if you only do very little exercise during the week. You will find that even with this approach, you can still lose a significant amount of weight.

The End Goal: Achieving Ketosis

The end goal for the Ketogenic Diet is the same for everyone: achieving that state of Ketosis. That's the time when your body is getting energy from the stored fat instead of the readily-available sugar you eat on a daily basis – but you know about that already.

The real question here is – how do you know you're *there?* Because weight loss in the Ketogenic Diet may be quick, but it's not *that* quick! You will be able to observe other changes even before the weight loss begins.

Chapter 6: Keto Side Effects and How to Solve Them

It would be very irresponsible of me if I only tell you all the good things about the Ketogenic Diet and ignore the side effects. The truth is that there are negative effects that could happen once you start the Ketogenic Diet – but that's actually true for all of them! All types of diet have negative effects to start with because your body has gotten used to the bad habits. Once you make the shift to a more positive way of eating, the body sort of goes on a rebellious phase so it feels like everything is going wrong. For example, a person who used to eat lots of sugar in a day can have severe headaches once they start to avoid the sugar. This is a withdrawal symptom and tells you that your diet is actually making positive changes to the body – albeit it takes a little bit of pain on your part.

So what can one expect when they make that change towards a healthy Ketogenic Diet? Here are some of the things to expect and of course – how to troubleshoot these problems.

Long Term Side Effects

A study titled *"Metabolic Effects of the Very Low Carbohydrate Diets: Misunderstood Villains of Human*

Metabolism" shows that for short-term purposes, the Ketogenic Diet is very effective. It lets you burn all those excess fat quickly but in a healthy way. If you do this for a long period of time however, there will be side effects. For example, there can be muscle loss, dizziness, kidney problems, acidosis, and problems with focus. Does that mean you shouldn't go on a Ketogenic Diet at all? Of course not! This only means that you'll have to be careful when using this diet. Don't push it too hard and you will be able to get all the positive results with none of the downsides!

Do you know why a low carbohydrate diet is bad if done for a long time? Well, balance is important in anything you do and the Ketogenic Diet doesn't really support balance. If you get rid of an entire food group for a long period of time, your body will rebel against you. Remember – the Ketogenic Diet relies on stored fat in your body. If there are no more stored fat, it really won't work anymore so you will have to increase your carbohydrates. To solve this problem, I recommend going on a 30-day Ketogenic Diet first and assessing your health before moving forward. Asking your doctor what to do "next" after the 30-day plan or after hitting your weight goal is also a good idea. Personally, I decided to increase my carbohydrate intake slightly after hitting my goal weight.

Keto Flu

The Keto Flu is the most prominent problem you'll encounter when starting the diet. It's a perfectly normal reaction by the body that may seem alarming because, well, the symptoms don't really feel good. You have to understand, your body has been running on a specific type of gasoline for years. It's been taking fuel from sugar and with the Ketogenic Diet, it's like you're changing your fuel source to a cleaner and more sustainable type. It makes sense that the engine growls a little in protest – but after that, you'll be able to run beautifully without the guilt.

The Keto Flu has the following symptoms:

- Headaches
- Fatigue
- Irritability
- Brain fog or difficulty focusing
- Motivational problems
- Sugar cravings
- Dizziness
- Nausea
- Muscle cramps
- Frequent urination

These symptoms are all heavily dependent on the kind of person doing the Keto Diet. Since you're already in our 50s, the symptoms may be more prominent, especially if you rely heavily on carbohydrates in your diet. If you eat mostly low-carb food however, these effects may not be as obvious.

But how do you solve them? Here are some of the best way to get rid of the Keto Flu as quickly as possible!

First, increase your water and salt consumption. This happens a lot once you start a Ketogenic Diet. You may not notice it, but a lot of the salt you consume is through carbohydrates like bread, pasta, rice, and so on. Salt tends to make you thirsty so if you eat little salt, you're also less likely to look for water during the day. So what happens now? Every time you feel dizzy or tired or nauseous while on a Keto Diet, just dissolve salt in water and gulp it down. Now, this is not going to taste good - but I promise that it will help you feel better. You can always try consuming the salt and water separately – whatever you find most convenient. Beef stock, bone broth, or chicken stock are also great alternatives and tastier too! I provided recipes for those in a later Chapter. As for water, try to hit a target of 3 liters of water every day. The good news is that this doesn't have to be plain water – your smoothies, coffee, and tea drinks are also counted.

Add more fat in your diet. Because of all the wrong information circulating today, a lot of people are afraid of fat. We've discussed this before but it bears repeating – fat is not your enemy. During the Ketogenic Diet, it makes sense to eat lots of fats especially if your carbohydrate intake dips to an all-time low. If you lower the carbohydrate consumption without an equal fat increase, then you will always feel hungry and tired.

Don't be impatient – go slower. Remember what we said about the body changing fuels when you're switching to the Ketogenic Diet? Well, the changing process doesn't have to be overnight. Choose to convert one meal at a time to a Keto-friendly set instead of changing all of them on your first day. Of course, it's recommended that you only do this if the salt water method doesn't for you. Just remember – the Keto Flu *will* pass so the first few days of discomfort should not discourage you in the slightest. If you want to minimize the trouble, try starting your Ketogenic Diet on a low-stress period – like a holiday. So basically, instead of eating less than 50 grams of carbohydrates a day, you can have a target of 50 to 70.

Do NOT count calories or restrict your food consumption. When it comes to the Ketogenic Diet – you don't have to calorie count. Again, you don't want to just stuff yourself with food just because you don't have to count calories, but the truth is calories do not matter so much when your body is at a state of Ketosis. It doesn't matter so much how many you're getting – your body will *always* break down the fat deposits and there will be weight loss. Stressing about the calorie intake or depriving yourself of food because of the calories can actually worsen the symptoms of Keto Flu and will make it more difficult for you to stick to the diet. The bottom line is this: as long as you're eating the allowed food items in allowed portions, then you're OK.

Limit your physical activity. That's the good news with the Ketogenic Diet – you don't have to exercise. Sure, you may not be running marathons or going to the gym on a weekly basis, but if you're health-conscious, then chances are you do light walks on a routine basis. That's perfectly OK – as long as you don't over-exert yourself. Now, there will be days when you will actually feel too good. Like you can go out and exercise because you have all this extra energy. When this happens, resist the temptation to do too much too soon. Your body is already burning as much fat as it can – don't push it too hard or you might get sick. If you're restless, try doing yoga, light walking, or just stretching.

Take some supplements. People using the Ketogenic Diet for a long time may also have vitamin and mineral deficiency. It's not easily obvious but it could happen so you'll have to be prepared. The usual vitamins and minerals lacking in a Ketogenic Diet include calcium, zinc, selenium, and vitamin D – so try taking a multivitamin during your diet. Again, I can't stress this enough: always consult your doctor before taking any sort of medication. This is especially true if you have pre-existing health problems and are also taking medication for maintenance.

Constipation or Diarrhea

These problems are fairly common because, well, you're changing your diet! Your body will react one way or another and in both cases, the solution is practically the same – water and fiber. Make sure you get enough fluids in your system and take fiber supplements which is available through many stores. You can also try taking laxatives that are made especially without carbohydrates.

If alarming symptoms occurs while you're on the Ketogenic Diet, I want you to consult your doctor ASAP! Again, reactions may vary from one person to the next and I don't want you shrugging off certain symptoms as if they're just "part" of the diet. Stay motivated but also be mindful of what is happening to your body. Remember – we want you to be healthy!

Chapter 7: Additional Things That Can Help

The Ketogenic Diet isn't as hard as it used to be thanks to the sudden popularity of the diet. For example, this book alone gives you dozens of ingredients to keep you satisfied even if you eat less carbohydrates. Aside from the basic Keto guidelines, here are additional sources of help to keep you going:

Keto Calculators

Not sure about the carbohydrate content of what you're eating? The good news is that there are Ketogenic Calculators today that should help you with the whole process! Thanks to the internet, you can go on your phone and search for the carb content of whatever you happen to be eating. The recipes provided in this book will also give you nutritional information and of course, there are some apps today that will give you Keto-friendly recipes complete with their nutritional content. Modern technology is a wonderful thing and can help you achieve ketosis!

Meal Plan Applications

The mobile phone is your friend. If you're having a tough time following a set meal plan or routine using the

Ketogenic Diet, you will find several online apps that can help. They're often free and will give you basic insight on how to proceed. While they're not ideal for the long haul, it can help you gain enough leverage to pursue this brand new lifestyle.

Ketone Test Strips

There are also these things called ketone test strips which are basically like pregnancy test kits or diabetes strips. They can be used to find out if you're already in that state of "ketosis" which means that your body is using the stored fat as fuel. Now, there are two types of ketone tests in the market today. The first one uses blood and the other uses urine.

Which one is more accurate? The blood of course! It works just like a diabetes indicator where you lance your finger, put some blood on the strip and insert it in a ketone meter. The meter will tell you if you're in a state of ketosis. This is the perfect measuring tool if you want to stick to ketosis for a long period of time.

Now, if you're perfectly new to the Ketogenic Diet, then the urine strips would be the better and more convenient option. It's not as accurate, but at least it doesn't require you to lance yourself. The only drawback of using urine strips is that they only work for the first few weeks of the Ketogenic

Diet. Why is that? Because during the first few weeks of the Ketogenic Diet, your body still isn't used to using the ketones. Hence, there's a high chance that your body will be disposing the ketones through urine. A high concentration of ketones in your urine tells you the diet is working. If you stick to the diet all through the 3rd and 4th week, the body becomes more used to using ketones. Hence, the ketone count during the 3rd and 4th week will be lower, so you'll actually have a faulty reading.

So to sum it up: urine ketone test strips are best used during your first and second weeks. After that, you can switch to blood strips or maybe just trust on the effectiveness of the diet and wait for the results!

List It Down

I want to encourage you to have some form of recording system. What does this mean? Simply put – I want you to have some kind of notebook or video or picture blog that can help you keep track of where you've been and where you're going. If you prefer the old-fashioned way of doing things, then you should thrive well with a notebook and a pen. Tracking your weight and writing down what you feel during a particular day will give you some insight on how the diet is doing for you. Plus, it can be an excellent source of motivation if you find yourself losing the drive to continue.

Chapter 8: Keto Grocery List

I've had people complain about the difficulty of switching their grocery list to one that's Ketogenic-friendly. The fact is that food is expensive – and most of the food you have in your fridge are probably packed full with carbohydrates. This is why if you're committing to a Ketogenic Diet, you need to do a clean sweep. That's right – everything that's packed with carbohydrates should be identified and set aside to make sure you're not eating more than you should. You can donate them to a charity before going out and buying your new Keto-friendly shopping list.

But what should be included in that list? The list really depends on what you want to eat. Fortunately, I have a wide range of Keto-friendly recipes in a later Chapter. Generally though, these are the food products you want to include in your cart:

Seafood

Seafood means fish like sardines, mackerel, and wild salmon. It's also a good idea to add some shrimp, tuna, mussels, and crab into your diet. This is going to be a tad expensive but definitely worth it in the long run. What's the common denominator in all these food items? The secret is omega-3 fatty acids which is credited for lots of health benefits. You want to add food rich in omega-3 fatty acids in your diet.

Low-carb Vegetables

Not all vegetables are good for you when it comes to the Ketogenic Diet. The vegetable choices should be limited to those with low carbohydrate counts. Pack up your cart with items like spinach, eggplant, arugula, broccoli, and cauliflower. You can also put in bell peppers, cabbage, celery, kale, Brussels sprouts, mushrooms, zucchini, and fennel.

So what's in them? Well, aside from the fact that they're low-carb, these vegetable also contain loads of fiber which makes digestion easier. Of course, there's also the presence of vitamins, minerals, antioxidants, and various other nutrients that you need for day to day life. Which ones should you avoid? Steer clear of the starch-packed vegetables like carrots, turnips, and beets. As a rule, you go for the vegetables that are green and leafy.

Fruits Low in Sugar

During an episode of sugar-craving, it's usually a good idea to pick low-sugar fruit items. Believe it or not, there are lots of those in the market! Just make sure to stock up on any of these: avocado, blackberries, raspberries, strawberries, blueberries, lime, lemon, and coconut. Also note that tomatoes are fruits too so feel free to make side dishes or dips with loads of tomatoes! Keep in mind that these fruits should be eaten fresh and not out of a can. If you do eat them fresh off the can however, take a good look at the nutritional information at the back of the packaging. Avocadoes are particularly popular for those practicing the Ketogenic Diet because they contains LOTS of the good kind of fat.

Meat and Eggs

While some diets will tell you to skip the meat, the Ketogenic Diet actually encourages its consumption. Meat is packed with protein that will feed your muscles and give you a consistent source of energy through the day. It's a slow but sure burn when you eat protein as opposed to carbohydrates which are burned faster and therefore stored faster if you don't use them immediately.

But what kind of meat should you be eating? There's chicken, beef, pork, venison, turkey, and lamb. Keep in mind that quality plays a huge role here – you should be eating grass-fed organic beef or organic poultry if you want to make the most out of this food variety. The organic option lets you limit the possibility of ingesting toxins in your body due to the production process of these products. Plus, the preservation process also means there are added salt or sugar in the meat, which can throw off the whole diet.

Nuts and Seeds

Nuts and seeds you should definitely add in your cart include: chia seeds, brazil nuts, macadamia nuts, flaxseed, walnuts, hemp seeds, pecans, sesame seeds, almonds, hazelnut, and pumpkin seeds. They also contain lots of protein and very little sugar so they're great if you have the munchies. They're the ideal snack because they're quick, easy, and will keep you full. They're high in calories though, which is why lots of people steer clear of them. As I mentioned earlier though – the Ketogenic Diet has nothing to do with calories and everything to do with the nutrient you're eating. So don't pay too much attention on the calorie count and just remember that they're a good source of fats and protein.

Dairy Products

OK – some people in their 50s already have a hard time processing dairy products, but for those who don't – you can happily add many of these to your diet. Make sure to consume sufficient amounts of cheese, plain Greek yogurt, cream butter, and cottage cheese. These dairy products are packed with calcium, protein, and the healthy kind of fat.

Oils

Nope, we're not talking about essentials oils but rather, MCT oil, coconut oil, avocado oil, nut oils, and even extra-virgin olive oil. You can start using those for your frying needs to create healthier food options. The beauty of these oils is that they add flavor to the food, making sure you don't get bored quickly with the recipes. Try picking up different types of Keto-friendly oils to add some variety to your cooking.

Coffee and Tea

The good news is that you don't have to skip coffee if you're going on a Ketogenic Diet. The bad news is that you can't go to Starbucks anymore and order their blended coffee choices. Instead, beverages would be limited to unsweetened tea or unsweetened coffee in order to keep the sugar consumption low. Opt for organic coffee and tea products to make the most out of these powerful antioxidants.

Dark Chocolate

Yes – chocolate is still on the menu, but it is limited to just dark chocolate. Technically, this means eating chocolate that is 70 percent cacao, which would make the taste a bit bitter.

Sugar Substitutes

Later in the recipes part of this book, you might be surprised at some of the ingredients required in the list. This is because while sweeteners are an important part of food preparation, you can't just use any kind of sugar in your recipe. Remember: the typical sugar is pure carbohydrate. Even if you're not eating carbohydrates, if you're dumping lots of sugar in your food – you're not really following the Ketogenic Diet principles.

So what do you do? You find sugar substitutes. The good news is that there are LOTS of those in the market. You can get rid of the old sugar and use any of these as a good substitute.

Stevia. This is perhaps the most familiar one in this list. It's a natural sweetener derived from plants and contains very few calories. Unlike your typical sugar, stevia may actually help lower the sugar levels instead of causing it to spike. Note though that it's sweeter than actual sugar so when cooking with stevia, you'll need to lower the amount used. Typically, the ratio is 200 grams of sugar per 1 teaspoon of powdered stevia.

Sucralose. It contains zero calories and zero carbohydrates. It's actually an artificial sweetener and does not metabolize – hence the complete lack of carbohydrates. Splenda is actually a sweetener derived from sucralose. Note though that you don't want to use this as a baking substitute for sugar. Its best use is for coffee, yogurt, and oatmeal sweetening. Note though that like stevia, it's also very sweet – in fact, it's actually 600 times sweeter than the typical sugar. Use sparingly.

Erythritol. It's a naturally occurring compound that interacts with the tongue's sweet taste receptors. Hence, it mimics the taste of sugar without actually being sugar. It does contain calories, but only about 5% of the calories you'll find in the typical sugar. Note though that it doesn't dissolve very well so anything prepared with this sweetener will have a gritty feeling. This can be problematic if you're using the product for baking. As for sweetness, the typical ratio is 1 1/3 cup for 1 cup of sugar.

Xylitol. Like erythritol, xylitol is a type of sugar alcohol that's commonly used in sugar-free gum. While it still contains calories, the calories are just 3 per gram. It's a sweetener that's good for diabetic patients because it doesn't raise the sugar levels or insulin in the body. The great thing about this is that you don't have to do any computations when using it for baking, cooking, or fixing a drink. The ratio of it with sugar is 1 to 1 so you can quickly make the substitution in the recipe.

What About Condiments?

Condiments are still on the table, but they won't be as tasty as you're used to. Your options include mustard, olive oil mayonnaise, oil-based salad dressings, and unsweetened ketchup. Of all these condiments, ketchup is the one with the most sugar, so make a point of looking for one with reduced sugar content. Or maybe avoid ketchup altogether and stick to mustard?

What About Snacks?

The good news is that there are packed snacks for those who don't have the time to make it themselves. Sugarless nut butters, dried seaweeds, nuts, and sugar-free jerky are all available in stores. The nuts and seeds discussed in a previous paragraph all make for excellent snack options.

What About Labels?

Let's not fool ourselves into thinking that we can cook food every single day. The fact is that there will be days when there will be purchases for the sake of convenience. There are also instances when you'll have problems finding the right ingredients for a given recipe. Hence, you'll need to find substitutes for certain ingredients without losing the "Keto friendly" vibe of the product.

So what should be done? Well, you need to learn how to read labels. Food doesn't have to be specially made to be keto-friendly, you just have to make sure that it doesn't contain any of the unfriendly nutrients or that the carbohydrate content is low enough.

Here's a step by step procedure on how to make a decision based on the labels:

1. First, take a good look at the ingredient list. You can usually find this at the bottom portion of the label and properly designated as "Ingredients".

2. The first step is to look at the sugar ingredient. If it's listed as one of the first five ingredients, then that already means there's too much sugar in the product to be keto friendly. Note though that sugar comes with many names. The words: glucose, fructose, maltose, lactose, dextrose, corn syrup and more, are all indicative of sugar content. You'd want to make sure they're not listed within the first 5 ingredients of the food product you're buying. That's one of the best things about the food industry – they're required to list ingredients in the order of quantity so that the first ones listed have more volume in the product.

3. If the food passes the "sugar" test, you should next look at the carbohydrate content.

4. You'll notice that carbohydrates are often broken down into groups. Hence, labels may indicate that total carbohydrates are 5grams and then right below that, you can see Dietary Fiber at 1gram and Sugar at 1gram. The important thing to note here is that the dietary fiber and the sugar are part of the total carbohydrates.

5. Why is this important? Well, most people count the total carbohydrates when computing their carbohydrate consumption for the day. Hence, if your goal is to eat less than 50grams of carbohydrates during the day, then you'll be computing using the 5gram amount.

6. Some people however make use of the "net carbohydrates" when computing their consumption. Net carbohydrates are what you get when you subtract the other carbohydrate sources from the total carbohydrates. Hence, 5 grams less 1 gram for the fiber and another gram for sugar mean that you'll have 3 grams of net carbohydrates.

7. Again – why is this important? The main distinction occurs for people who have diabetes. It's all about the insulin levels. At the end of the day however, it's all about the 50 grams of carbohydrates limitation in your diet. If you want to stay on the safe side

however, then counting the total carbohydrates is usually the best option.

8. Look at the serving size. Most people think that the nutrition information in the packet refers to all the food items in the pack – but that's not the case at all. The nutritional information is per serving so you'd want to make sure that the carbohydrate content you picture in your head is equal to the food you usually eat in one sitting. For example, a packet of nuts contains 5 serving in total, each serving containing around 5 grams of carbohydrates. If you eat 2 servings in one sitting, then you'll have to remember that you're consuming 10 grams instead of just 5.

Once you've figured this out, you can quickly make calculations in your head about carbohydrate content of what you're eating based on the labels. You will find that this can be easily adjusted to your eating habits so that you always know what you're consuming even if you're not following a set recipe.

Chapter 9: Simple Keto Recipes

The beauty of the Ketogenic Diet is that there are numerous recipes available today to help you get started. In this Chapter, I'll walk you through some of the more popular Keto recipes available today and the nutritional information each one has to help guide you through the process.

Keto Breakfast Recipes

Banana Waffles

Cooking Time: 30 minutes

Servings: 4 servings

Ingredient List:

- 4 eggs
- 1 ripe banana
- ¾ cup coconut milk
- ¾ cup almond flour
- 1 pinch of salt
- 1 tbsp. of ground psyllium husk powder
- ½ tsp. vanilla extract
- 1 tsp. baking powder

- 1 tsp. of ground cinnamon
- Butter or coconut oil for frying

Instructions:

1. Mash the banana thoroughly until you get a mashed potato consistency.
2. Add all the other ingredients in and whisk thoroughly to evenly distribute the dry and wet ingredients. You should be able to get a pancake-like consistency
3. Fry the waffles in a pan or use a waffle maker.
4. You can serve it with hazelnut spread and fresh berries. Enjoy!

Nutrition Facts: each waffle contains 4g of carbohydrates, 13g fat, 5g protein, and 155 kcalories

Keto Cinnamon Coffee

Cooking Time: 5 minutes

Servings: 1 serving

Ingredient List:

- 2 tbsp. ground coffee
- 1/3 cup heavy whipping cream
- 1 tsp. ground cinnamon
- 2 cups water

Instructions:

1. Start by mixing the cinnamon with the ground coffee.
2. Pour in hot water and do what you usually do when brewing.
3. Use a mixer or whisk to whip the cream 'til you get stiff peaks
4. Serve in a tall mug and put the whipped cream on the surface. Sprinkle with some cinnamon and enjoy.

Nutrition Facts: 1 gram net carbs, 1 gram fiber, 14 grams fat, 1 gram protein, 136kcalories

Keto Waffles and Blueberries

*Cooking Time:*10 to 15 minutes

Servings: 8

Ingredient List:

- 8 eggs
- 5 oz. melted butter
- 1 tsp. vanilla extract
- 2 tsp. baking powder
- 1/3 cup coconut flour
- 3 oz. butter (topping)
- 1 oz. fresh blueberries (topping)

Instructions:

1. Start by mixing the butter and eggs first until you get a smooth batter. Put in the remaining ingredients except those that we'll be using as topping.
2. Heat your waffle iron to medium temperature and start pouring in the batter for cooking
3. In a separate bowl, mix the butter and blueberries using a hand mixer. Use this to top off your freshly cooked waffles

Nutrition Facts: 3g net carbs, 5g fiber, 56g fat, 14g protein, and 575 kcalories

Baked Avocado Eggs

Cooking Time: 30 minutes maximum

Servings: 4 servings

Ingredient List:

- 2 avocados
- 4 eggs
- ½ cup bacon bits, around 55 grams
- 2 tbsp. fresh chives, chopped
- 1 sprig of chopped fresh basil, chopped
- 1 cherry tomato, quartered

- Salt and pepper to taste
- Shredded cheddar cheese

Instructions:

1. Start by preheating the oven to 400 degrees Fahrenheit
2. Slice the avocado and remove the pits. Put them on a baking sheet and crack some eggs onto the center hole of the avocado. If it's too small, just scoop out more of the flesh to make room. Salt and pepper to taste.
3. Top with bacon bits and bake for 15 minutes.
4. Remove and sprinkle with herbs. Enjoy!

Nutrition Facts: Contains around 271 calories, 21g of fat, 7g fat, 5g fiber, 13g protein, and 7g carbohydrates

Mushroom Omelet

Cooking Time: 5 minutes

Servings: 1 serving

Ingredient List:

- 3 eggs, medium
- 1 oz. shredded cheese
- 1 oz. butter used for frying

- ¼ yellow onion, chopped
- 4 large sliced mushrooms
- Your favorite vegetables, optional
- Salt and pepper to taste

Instructions:

1. Crack and whisk the eggs in a bowl. Add some salt and pepper to taste.
2. Melt the butter in a pan using low heat. Put in the mushroom and onion, cooking the two until you get that amazing smell.
3. Pour the egg mix into the pan and allow it to cook on medium heat.
4. Allow the bottom part to cook before sprinkling the cheese on top of the still-raw portion of the egg.
5. Carefully pry the edges of the omelet and fold it in half. Allow it to cook for a few more seconds before removing the pan from the heat and sliding it directly onto your plate.

Nutrition Facts: 5 grams of carbohydrates. 1 gram of fiber, 44 grams of fat, 26 grams of protein, and 520 kcalories

Soft Boiled Keto Eggs

Cooking Time: 15 minutes

Servings: 1 serving

Ingredient List:

- 3 large eggs
- 1 tbsp. of unsalted butter
- ¼ tsp. thyme leaves
- Freshly ground black pepper
- Salt to taste

Instructions:

1. Grab a saucepan and fill it halfway with water, apply high heat until the water boils.
2. When boiling, gently place the eggs in the water. Set a timer for 6 minutes.
3. Take on tablespoon of butter and put it in the microwave for around 20 seconds or until it melts.
4. Remove the eggs from the saucepan, carefully pouring the hot water in the sink. This is great because the hot water can also help remove clogs from your pipes!
5. Carefully take a bowl and fill it with cold water. Put the eggs inside so it can cool off. Once done, peel the egg and place it in your bowl of melted butter.

6. Add salt and pepper to taste and thyme for garnishing. Make sure to eat it while fresh!

Nutrition Facts: 340 kcalories,

French Omelet

Cooking Time: 20 to 25 minutes

Servings: 2 servings

Ingredient List:

- 2 large eggs
- 4 large egg whites
- ¼ cup fat-free milk
- ¼ cup cubed ham, cooked
- ¼ cup cheddar cheese, shredded
- 1/8 tsp. salt
- 1/8 tsp. pepper
- 1 tbsp. onion, chopped
- 1 tbsp. green pepper, chopped

Instructions:

1. Whisk together the eggs and egg whites until blended.
2. Add the salt, pepper, and milk, mixing them together until fully blended.

3. Using medium heat, coat your skillet with cooking spray and pour the egg mixture in when the surface is hot and ready.

4. As it cooks, push it around the edges so the uncooked portion flows around until there are no runny liquid on top.

5. When it's already around ¾ cooked, put all the remaining ingredients on top and continue cooking until done.

Nutrition Facts: Per serving there's around 186 calories, 9 grams of fat, 4 grams carbohydrate, 22 grams protein, 648 mg of sodium and 207 mg of cholesterol.

Apple Chicken Sausage

Cooking Time: 25 to 30 minutes

Servings: 8 patties

Ingredient List:

- 1 large tart apple, diced
- 1 pound ground chicken
- ¼ tsp. pepper
- 1 tsp. salt
- 2 tsp. poultry seasoning

Instructions:

1. Grab a large bowl and combine all the ingredients except the ground chicken

2. Combine the chicken in the mix and blend well. Create a total of 8 patties of similar sizes which should be around 3 inches in diameter each.

3. Cook them up using medium heat. Make sure each side gets around 5 to 6 minutes of cooking time.

Nutrition Facts: each sausage patty contains 92 calories, 5 grams of fat, 9 grams of protein, 4 grams of carbohydrates, 1 gram of fiber, 38 mg of cholesterol, and 328 mg of sodium.

Keto Cereal

Cooking Time: 1 hour and 15 minutes

Servings: 12 servings

Ingredient List:

- 1 cup shredded coconut, unsweetened
- 1 cup flaked coconut, unsweetened
- ½ cup flaxseeds
- ½ cup flaked almonds
- 1/3 cup Pepitas
- 1/3 cup sunflower seeds

- 1/3 cup chia seeds
- 1/3 cup erythritol
- 1/3 cup melted coconut oil
- 1 tbsp. ground cinnamon
- 1 tsp. vanilla extract

Instructions:

- Preheat your over to 150 degrees Celsius or 300 degrees Fahrenheit
- Mix all the ingredients together in one convenient bowl.
- Once they're combined, spread them over a pan on top of a lined cookie sheet
- Bake them for 25 to 35 minutes. You might have to take them out every five minutes and stir up the mix to prevent burning.
- The goal is to create an even golden brown or have them reach that lightly toasted color. Once you've got that, remove them from the oven.
- Allow to cool and break them up and store in an airtight container.

Nutrition Facts: each serving should contain 244 kcalories, 9 grams of carbohydrates, 4 grams of protein, 22 grams of fat, 8 mg of sodium, 195 mg of potassium, 6 grams of fiber, 1 gram of sugar.

Keto Breakfast Burrito

Cooking Time: 10 minutes

Servings: 1 serving

Ingredient List:

- 1 tbsp butter
- 2 eggs medium
- 2 tbsp full fat cream
- choice of herbs or spices
- salt and pepper to taste

Instructions:

1. Grab a bowl and whisk the eggs and cream together. Add your choice of herbs and spices, depending on personal preferences.
2. Melt the butter in a frying pan using low to medium heat.
3. Pour the egg mixture into the pan.
4. Cook and swirl to create a thin layer of egg burrito.
5. Gently lift the egg burrito from the frying pan. Put the fillings you want inside and roll it up. Enjoy!

Nutrition Facts: 331 calories, 30g fat, 1g carbohydrates, and 11g protein.

Keto Lunch Recipes

Low Carb Keto Meatloaf

Cooking Time: 60 minutes

Servings: 6 servings

Ingredient List:

- 2 lbs 85% lean grass fed ground beef
- 2 large eggs
- 4 cloves garlic
- 1/2 tbsp fine salt
- 2 tbsp avocado oil
- 1 tbsp lemon zest
- 1 tsp black pepper
- 1/4 cup nutritional yeast
- 1/4 cup chopped parsley
- 1/4 cup chopped fresh oregano

Instructions:

1. Preheat oven to 400 degrees Fahrenheit
2. Grab a bowl and put in the beef, salt, nutritional yeast, and black pepper
3. In a separate bowl, mix the eggs, herbs, garlic, and oil. Blend them together until you get a really

frothy mixture. It's best to use a blender for this so that the other ingredients come out minced and fully mixed.

4.   Combine the egg blend and beef.

5.   Put the beef mixture in a loaf pan. Smoothen it out.

6.   Place on the middle rack and bake for 60 minutes.

7.   Remove and allow it to drain. Let cool for the next 10 minutes

8.   Served best with fresh lemon.

Nutrition Facts: contains 344 calories, 29g fat, 2g fiber, 33g protein, and 4g carbohydrates.

Grilled Cedar Plan Salmon Burgers

Cooking Time: 30 minutes

Servings: 4 servings

Ingredient List:

- 1 stalk celery, diced
- 1 ½ lbs wild caught salmon fillets
- 1 ½ tbsp mayonnaise
- 1 ½ tbsp mustard
- 2 tbsp fresh dill

- 2 cloves garlic, minced
- 2 tsp salt
- 1 tsp black pepper
- ½ small red onion, diced
- Fresh lemon juice, to taste

Instructions:

1.　　Soak the cedar planks for 2 hours in water.

2.　　Preheat the grill to 350 degrees Fahrenheit

3.　　Remove the skin and bones from the salmon. Cut it up into smaller pieces and put in the food processor.

4.　　Add mayo, mustard, pepper, salt, and garlic in the processor and pulse several times until you get a smooth paste.

5.　　Scrap the paste and put it in a mixing bowl. Put the onion and celery and mix thoroughly.

6.　　Put the planks on the grill and let them preheat.

7.　　While waiting, form the salmon mixture into patties.

8.　　Grill the patties on the plan for 30 minutes each side or until you're satisfied that it's cooked all the way through.

9.　　Serve with squeezed lemon top

Nutrition Facts: contains 360 calories, 16.76g fat, 1.7g net carbohydrates, and 47g protein

Keto Egg Salad

Cooking Time: 30 minutes

Servings: 2 servings

Ingredient List:

- 1 avocado
- 6 eggs
- 1/3 cup mayonnaise
- 1 tsp Dijon mustard
- Splash of lemon juice to prevent avocado from browning
- Salt & pepper to taste

Instructions:

1. Put water in a saucepan and bring to boil. Put the eggs inside it and turn off the heat. The hot water will cook the egg for the next 10 to 15 minutes.

2. Put the egg in cold water. Allow it to cool before peeling the shells.

3. Chop the eggs and sprinkle with salt & pepper to taste. Set it aside.

4.   Mash the avocado and season it with salt & pepper as well.

5.   Grab a bowl and mix the eggs, mashed avocado, and mayonnaise together. Put in the lemon juice, mustard, and the herbs you want.

6.   Chill and serve.

Nutrition Facts: 575 calories, 51g fat, 7g carbohydrates, 5g fiber, and 2g protein.

Keto Chicken Bacon Cheese Wraps

Cooking Time: 7 minutes

Servings: 2 servings

Ingredient List:

- 6 mozzarella cheese slices
- 2 cheddar cheese slices
- 1 tbsp ranch
- 2 tbsp Guacamole
- ½ cup cooked chicken
- ¼ cup Lettuce
- 4 cooked bacon

Instructions:

1.   Start by preheating the oven to 375 degrees Fahrenheit. Prepare your baking pan with parchment paper.

2.   Spread the 6 slices of cheese on the pan with the edges touching each other.

3.   Bake the cheese for 4 to 5 minutes or until the edges turn brown. This will give you cheese tortilla

4.   Let it cool down before placing the guacamole on the edges of the cheese wrap. Spread the lettuce on the guacamole.

5.   Cover the guacamole with the cooked bacon and chicken. Cover it all with the cheddar slices.

6.   Spread the dressing on the other end of the wrap. This will be like the glue of the wrap as you tightly roll it around.

Nutrition Facts: each wrap is worth 2 servings, each serving containing 450 calories, 30.6g fat, 1.9g carbohydrates, 42.5g protein, and 0.8g fiber

Stuffed Peppers

Cooking Time: 30 minutes

Servings: 6 servings

Ingredient List:

- 1½ cups marinara sauce
- 6 bell peppers
- 1 lb 4 oz ground beef
- 1 tsp paprika
- ½ tsp dried oregano
- ½ tsp ground mustard
- 1 sweet onion, minced
- 2 garlic cloves, minced
- ¾ cup cooked rice
- ¼ cup chopped fresh parsley
- ½ cup shredded Jack cheese
- Salt and freshly ground black pepper

Instructions:

1.   Start by preheating the oven to 375 degrees Fahrenheit.

2.   Prepare the oven-safe skillet by pouring marinara sauce on the base.

3.   Cut off the top of the pepper and remove the ribs and seeds, leaving it completely empty.

4.   Grab a bowl and mix the onion, rice, paprika, garlic, oregano, mustard, and beef together. Stir thoroughly before adding the parsley, salt, and pepper to taste. Combine thoroughly to properly distribute the flavor.

5.   Stuff the meat mixture into each pepper all the way up to the rim.

6.   Put the peppers in the skillet, making sure they're standing up on the rack.

7.   Garnish with 1 ½ tbsp of cheese on top.

8.   Bake for 25 minutes or until the pepper becomes tender.

9.   Serve with sauce as soon as its cooked. This doesn't keep for long so try to eat it as soon as it's done.

Nutrition Facts: each serving contains 166 calories, 23g carbohydrates, 6g protein, and 5g fat

Keto Chicken Casserole

Cooking Time: 20 to 30 minutes

Servings: 1 serving

Ingredient List:

- 2 tbsp. heavy whipping cream
- 1/10 cup cream cheese
- 1/10 lemon juice
- ½ tbsp. green pesto
- ¼ oz. butter
- 1/3 lb. skinless, boneless chicken cut into small pieces

- 1/6 leek, chopped
- 1/6 lb. cauliflower, cut
- Salt & pepper to taste
- 2/3 oz cherry tomatoes, halved
- 1 ¼ oz. shredded cheese

Instructions:

1. Start by preheating the oven to 400 degrees Fahrenheit
2. Mix the cream and cream cheese together with the lemon juice and pesto. Use the salt & pepper to taste. Set aside.
3. Using medium heat, melt the butter in a large pan. Put in the seasoned chicken and fry until you get that nice golden brown color.
4. Once done, put the greased chicken in a baking dish and place the creamy mixture on the chicken.
5. Top off the chicken with the tomatoes, leek, and cauliflower. Sprinkle some cheese on top and bake it for 30 minutes.
6. Remove and enjoy!

Nutrition Facts: contains 739 kcalories, 37g protein, 2g fiber, 62g fat, and 7g net carbohydrates

Lasagna Stuffed Portobello's

Cooking Time: 1 hour to 1 hour and 30 minutes

Servings: 4 servings

Ingredient List:

- 4 portobello mushrooms, large
- 12 oz. of ground meat of your choice
- 1 cup sugar free marinara sauce
- 1 cup whole milk shredded mozzarella cheese
- 1 cup whole milk ricotta cheese
- Chopped parsley for garnishing

Instructions:

1. Preheat your oven to 375 degrees Fahrenheit
2. Start cleaning the mushrooms by removing stems as well as scraping brown portions along the ribs.
3. Stuff the meat inside the mushrooms until well packed.
4. Pack in around ¼ cup of ricotta into the mushroom cup and press, leaving just enough room in the center where the sauce will be placed
5. Spoon in the ¼ cup of marinara on the top. Finally, sprinkle some mozzarella cheese on top of the mushroom
6. Bake for 40 minutes. Garnish with parsley after removing from the oven. Enjoy!

Nutrition Facts: each portobello is one serving with a total of 482 calories, 36 grams of fat, around 6.5 grams of carbohydrates, and 28 grams of protein.

Keto Baked Salmon with Lemon Butter

Cooking Time: 25 to 30 minutes

Servings: 6 servings

Ingredient List:

- 1 lemon, thinly sliced
- 1 tbsp. olive oil
- 2 lbs. salmon
- 1 tsp. sea salt
- 7 oz. butter, thinly sliced
- Ground black pepper

Instructions:

1. Preheat the oven to 400 degrees Fahrenheit
2. Grease the baking dish with olive oil and put the salmon on the surface. Make sure to put it skin-side down. Season with salt & pepper to taste.
3. Place the thinly sliced lemons on the salmon and cover it with the butter.

4. Place in the middle rack and back for 30 minutes or until the salmon turns flaky.

5. Grab some more butter and heat it in a sauce pan. Put some lemon juice in the mix and serve beside the tuna. Enjoy!

Nutrition Facts: contains 1g of carbohydrates, 49g fat, 573 kcalories, and 31g protein

Keto Chicken and Cabbage Plate

Cooking Time: 5 to 10 minutes

Servings: 2 servings

Ingredient List:

- 7 oz. fresh green cabbage, shredded
- 1 lb. rotisserie chicken
- ½ red onion
- ½ cup mayonnaise
- 1 tbsp. olive oil
- Salt & pepper

Instructions:

1. Thinly slice the onions and combine it with the shredded cabbage in a plate.

2. Add the rotisserie chicken in the plate and put a tablespoon of mayonnaise on the side

3. Drizzle some olive oil, salt, and pepper to taste. Enjoy!

Nutrition Facts: Contains 1041kcalories, 48g protein, 7g net carbohydrates, 91g fat, and 3g fiber

Keto Chicken Recipe

Cooking Time: 30 minutes

Servings: 4 servings

Ingredient List:

- 8 medium sized uncooked chicken breast tenders
- 24-oz pickle jar
- 2 scoops of 100% whey protein powder, unflavored
- ¼ cup grated parmesan
- 2 tbsp avocado oil
- 1 tsp paprika
- 2 large eggs
- Salt & pepper to taste

Instructions:

1.   Put chicken in a plastic bag and pour the pickles inside. Put a lid on it and allow the chicken to marinate in the pickle.

2.   In the meantime, mix together the protein powder, salt, pepper, paprika, and grated parmesan.

3.   Crack the eggs in a separate bowl and beat thoroughly.

4.   Preheat the skillet. Put the avocado oil on the pan.

5.   While heating up the oil, dip the chicken tender in the egg. When done, coat it with the bread mixture.

6.   Fry the chicken until golden brown and fully cooked.

Nutrition Facts: 342.53 calories, 14.8g fats, 1.68g net carbohydrates and 47.6g protein.

Ginger Mackerel Lunch Bowl

Cooking Time: 30 to 45 minutes

Servings: 2 servings

Ingredient List:

- 1 tbsp grated ginger (marinade)
- 1 tbsp lemon juice (marinade)

- 3 tbsp olive oil (marinade)
- 1 tbsp coconut aminos (marinade)
- Salt & pepper, to taste (marinade)
- 8 oz boneless mackerel fillets (lunch bowl)
- 1 oz almonds (lunch bowl)
- 1 ½ cups broccoli (lunch bowl)
- 1 tbsp butter (lunch bowl)
- ½ small yellow onion (lunch bowl)
- 1/3 cup diced red bell pepper (lunch bowl)
- 2 small sun-dried tomatoes, chopped (lunch bowl)
- 4 tbsp mashed avocado (lunch bowl)

Instructions:

1.   Preheat the oven to 400 degrees Fahrenheit.

2.   In a bowl, combine the grated ginger, olive oil, lemon juice, coconut aminos, salt & pepper. Rub half of the marinade on the mackerel fillets.

3.   Line the baking tray with parchment paper. Place the mackerel fillets with the skin side facing upwards.

4.   Roast it for 12 to 15 minutes until it gets crispy

5.   On a separate baking sheet, roast the almonds for 5 minutes until they turn brown. Allow them to cool down before chopping it up. Set aside.

6.   Steam the broccoli to soften it up before chopping.

7.   Preheat the pan using medium heat. Melt the butter and fry the onions and pepper until they become soft.

8.   Put the sun dried tomatoes and broccoli and cook.

9.   When done, turn the heat off and the roasted almonds and the rest of the dressing.

10.   Serve it with avocado.

Nutrition Facts: 649.55 calories, 53 fats, 9g net carbohydrates, and 28g protein

Keto Baking Recipes

Keto Chocolate Chip Cookies

Cooking Time: 50 minutes

Servings: 12 cookies

Ingredient List:

- 1 egg
- 3.5 oz salted butter
- 4.5 oz erythritol
- 3 oz sugar free chocolate chips
- 6 oz almond flour

- 1 tsp vanilla extract
- 1/2 tsp baking powder
- 1/4 tsp salt

Instructions:

- Start by preheating the oven to 355 degrees Fahrenheit
- Microwave the butter for 30 seconds to melt.
- Combine the melted butter with the erythritol and beat thoroughly.
- Add the egg and vanilla. Mix it again for 15 seconds.
- Put in the baking powder, almond flour, salt, and xantham gum. Beat until fully combined.
- Press the dough together and knead. Add the chocolate chips.
- Divide into 12 balls and arrange it on the baking tray. Bake for 10 minutes.
- Let it cool before serving. Enjoy!

Nutrition Facts: contains 168kcalories, 17.3g fat, 2.3g carbohydrates, 4g protein.

Basic Keto Bread

Cooking Time: 55 minutes

Servings: 16 slices

Ingredient List:

- 7 eggs
- 1 tsp baking powder
- 1/2 tsp xantham gum
- 1/2 tsp salt
- 3.5 oz melted butter
- 1 oz coconut oil
- 7 oz almond flour

Instructions:

1. Preheat the oven to 355 degrees Fahrenheit
2. Crack and beat the eggs for 2 minutes or until foamy.
3. Put in the melted butter, xantham gum, salt, and baking powder. Beat it until the mixture becomes thick
4. Put it in a loaf pan prepped with baking paper. Bake for 45 minutes
5. Slice into 16 thin slices. Store this in an airtight container in the fridge. It should last for up to 7 days.

Nutrition Facts: 165kcalories per slice, 15g fat, 4.8g saturated fat, 3g carbohydrates, 6g protein, and 1.5g fiber

Keto Lemon Bars

Cooking Time: 60 minutes

Servings: 8 servings

Ingredient List:

- 3 lemons
- 3 eggs
- 1/2 cup melted butter
- 1 3/4 cups almond flour, divided
- 1 cup powdered erythritol, divided

Instructions:

1. Preheat the oven to 350 degrees Fahrenheit
2. Mix the butter, a pinch of salt, 1 cup almond flour, and ¼ cup erythritol in a bowl.
3. Put the resulting mixture into a prepared baking dish.
4. Cook for 20 minutes. Let it cool for 20 minutes.
5. While cooling, juice all the lemons in a bowl and zest one of them. Add the eggs, ¾ cup almond flour, ¾ cup erythritol, and just a pinch of salt. Combine it thoroughly. This will be your filling.
6. Pour the filling on the crust and bake for 25 more minutes
7. Serve with a sprinkle of erythritol on top. Enjoy!

Nutrition Facts: per bar contains about 272 calories, 26g fat, 46 carbohydrates, 8g protein

Easy Keto Butter Cake Recipe

Cooking Time: 2 hours 40 minutes

Servings: 10 slices

Ingredient List:

- 2 large eggs
- 3 tbsp coconut flour
- 1 tsp baking powder
- 8 tbsp butter
- 1/4 cup powdered erythritol
- 1/2 tsp vanilla extract
- 8 tbsp butter, room temperature (top layer)
- 8 oz cream cheese, room temperature (top layer)
- 1/4 cup powdered erythritol (top layer)
- 1/2 tsp vanilla extract (top layer)
- 50 drops liquid stevia (top layer)
- 2 large eggs, room temperature (top layer)

Instructions:

1. Start by preheating your oven to 350 degrees. While waiting, grease an 8-inch springform pan sprayed with coconut oil.
2. We're starting with the bottom layer first. Combine the butter, eggs, and vanilla extract in a mixing bowl and whisk them all together thoroughly.

3. Put in the erythritol, coconut flour, and baking powder. Blend and set aside.

4. We'll start with the bottom layer next. Put together the cream, cream cheese, and butter. Mix it together in a large mixing bowl.

5. Put in the vanilla, erythritol, eggs, and stevia. Combine until smooth.

6. Put in the bottom layer mixture into the springform pan. This will be the cake's crust.

7. Next, pour the top layer slowly. Make sure to tap the pan a few times to prevent bubbles from forming.

8. Bake for 30 to 35 minutes.

9. When the sides are browning, take it out of the oven and allow it to cool. This should take 15 to 20 minutes.

Nutrition Facts: 1 slice will have 295 calories, 30g total fat, 9g cholesterol, 2g carbohydrates, 1g sugar, 5g protein.

Low Carb Keto Cupcake Recipe

Cooking Time: 35 minutes

Servings: 12 cupcakes

Ingredient List:

- 4 eggs

- 1/3 cup coconut flour
- ½ cup unsweetened cocoa powder
- ¼ cup powdered erythritol
- 1 tsp. baking powder
- ½ tsp baking soda
- ¼ tsp. salt
- 1 tsp. vanilla extract
- 4 tbsp. extra light olive oil
- ½ cup unsweetened almond milk

Instructions:

1. Start by preheating oven the 350 degrees Fahrenheit. Grab the muffin tin and grease is up or put the cupcake liners while waiting.

2. Grab a bowl and combine the cocoa powder, coconut flour, baking powder, baking soda, salt, and erythritol. Whisk all the ingredients thoroughly.

3. Add the eggs, vanilla extract, almond oil, and olive oil. Mix completely until they're well combined. Allow it to sit for 5 minutes. Check to see if the mixture has the desired thickness. If not, you can add water until gets the thickness you want. Make sure to add one tablespoon at a time to help control the amount.

4. Put around 2 tablespoons of the batter into the muffin tin.

5. Bake for 20 minutes or until a toothpick comes out clean after inserting it in the center of the muffin.

Nutrition Facts: contains 66 kcalories, 45g fat, 16g saturated fat, 1mg cholesterol, 88mg potassium, 2g fiber, and 1g protein.

Chocolate Keto Cake

Cooking Time: 15 to 20 minutes

Servings: 8 servings

Ingredient List:

- 3 eggs
- 2 tbsp. Dutch cocoa
- 1 ½ tsp. pure vanilla extract
- 1 ½ cups fine almond flour
- ¼ cup cocoa powder
- 1/3 cup water or milk
- 1/3 cup regular sugar
- 2 ¼ tsp. baking powder
- ½ tsp. salt

Instructions:

1. Preheat the oven to 350 degrees Fahrenheit. While waiting, grease an 8-inch pan.

2. Combine the ingredients and stir well before putting it in the pan. Smooth the top surface and jiggle the pan a little to get rid of any possible air pockets inside.

3. Put the pan on the center rack and bake for 14 minutes. Make sure it's completely cooked before you put frosting.

Nutrition Facts: Contains 130 calories, 2.7g of net carbohydrates, 9g of fat, 175mg of sodium, and 3.3g of dietary fiber.

Keto Avocado Brownies

Cooking Time: 45 to 60 minutes

Servings: 16 servings

Ingredient List:

- 4 large eggs
- 2 ripe avocado
- ½ cup melted butter
- 6 tbsp. unsweetened peanut butter
- 2 tsp. baking soda
- 2 tsp. pure vanilla extract
- ½ tsp. kosher salt

- 2/3 cup granulated sugar, preferably keto-friendly
- 2/3 cup cocoa powder, unsweetened

Instructions:

1. Start by preheating the oven to 350 degrees.
2. Grab a square pan and line it with parchment paper.
3. Take a blender and just dump all the ingredients inside it. Blend until smooth. If you have a food processor, you can use that too.
4. Transfer the batter onto the pan, smoothing out the surface with a spatula
5. Bake the brownies for 25 to 30 minutes or until the brownies are soft and firm. Allow to cool before serving

Nutrition Facts: 260 calories per serving, with 7 grams of protein, 11 grams carbohydrates, 5 grams fiber, 1 gram sugar, 23 grams fat, 9 grams saturated fat, and around 570mg of sodium.

Keto Fudge

Cooking Time: 15 to 20 minutes

Serving Size: 12

Ingredient List

- 1 cup coconut oil, soft but still sold

- ¼ cup full fat coconut milk

- ¼ cup Swerve confectioners

- ¼ cup organic cocoa powder

- 1 tsp. vanilla extract

- ½ tsp. Celtic sea salt

- ½ tsp. almond extract

Instructions:

1. Combine the coconut oil and coconut milk in a bowl and mix them together for 6 minutes or until you get that glossy well-mixed texture.

2. Put in all the remaining ingredients and stir, going slow first and then slowly increasing it so that the cocoa doesn't wind up all over the kitchen counter.

3. Taste the resulting mixture and just add in ingredients depending on your favored sweetness.

4. Pour them all in small molds or put them in a pan lined with wax paper. Store them in the freezer for just 15 minutes to solidify the whole thing up.

5. Cut them up and put them in a container ready to be served. Remember, you'll have to store them in the fridge or the mix will liquefy.

Nutrition Facts: contains170 Calories, 19 grams Fat, 1 gram Protein, 1 gram fiber,

Keto Cookies

Cooking Time: 45 minutes to 1 hour

Servings: 15 cookies

Ingredient List:

- 4 egg yolks, large
- 3 tbsp. of butter
- ½ tsp. kosher salt
- 1 cup coconut flakes
- 1 cup sugar free dark chocolate chips
- ¼ cup of coconut oil
- ¾ cup walnuts, chopped
- 3 tbsp. of granulated Swerve sweetener

Instructions:

1. Start by preheating your oven to 350 degrees. Prepare your baking sheet by lining it with parchment paper.
2. Grab a large bowl and put in the coconut oil, sweetener, salt, butter, and egg yolks. Mix them all together until you get a creamy consistency. Add the

chocolate chips, coconut, and walnuts and mix it some more.

3. Drop the resulting mix onto the baking sheet, one spoonful glob at a time.

4. Bake them for 15 minutes or until golden. Enjoy!

Nutrition Facts: 130 calories per serving, 2 grams of protein, 1 gram of fiber, 13 grams of fat, 8 grams of saturated fat, 25 mg of sodium, and 2 grams of carbohydrates.

Keto Vanilla Pound Cake

Cooking Time: 1 hour 5 minutes

Servings: 12 servings

Ingredient List:

- 4 large eggs
- Top of Form
- Bottom of Form
- 2 cups almond flour
- 1 cup erythritol
- 1 cup sour cream
- 1/2 cup butter
- 2 tsp baking powder
- 1 tsp vanilla extract

- 2 ounces cream cheese

Instructions:

1. Start by preheating the oven to 350 degrees Fahrenheit
2. Butter a 9 inch pan for the baking
3. Grab a large bowl and put the flour and baking powder inside.
4. Cut the butter into squares and add cream cheese. Microwave it for 30 seconds to melt both. Stir until they're well combined
5. Add the erythritol sweetener, sour cream, and vanilla extract to the mix of butter and cream cheese.
6. Combine the wet ingredients with the dry ingredients.
7. Crack the eggs open and beat thoroughly. Add them to the other ingredients and stir complete.
8. Pour the batter into the pan and bake for 50 minutes. Make sure the cake cools for 2 hours before serving.

Nutrition Facts: Each serving contains 249 calories, 20.67g fat, 5.2g carbohydrates, and 7.67 protein

Keto Dinner Recipes

Keto Sloppy Joes

Cooking Time: 30 to 45 minutes

Servings: 1 serving

Ingredient List:

- 1 ¼ cup almond flour (for the bread)
- 5 tbsp. ground psyllium husk powder (for the bread)
- 1 tsp. sea salt (for the bread)
- 2 tsp. baking powder (for the bread)
- 2 tsp. cider vinegar (for the bread)
- 1 ¼ cups boiling water (for the bread)
- 3 egg whites (for the bread)
- 2 tbsp. olive oil (for the meat sauce)
- 1 ½ lbs. ground beef (for the meat sauce)
- 1 yellow onion (for the meat sauce)
- 4 garlic clover (for the meat sauce)
- 14 oz. crushed tomatoes (for the meat sauce)
- 1 tbsp. chili powder (for the meat sauce)
- 1 tbsp. Dijon powder (for the meat sauce)
- 1 tbsp. red wine vinegar (for the meat sauce)
- 4 tbsp. tomato paste (for the meat sauce)
- 2 tsp. salt (for the meat sauce)
- ¼ tsp ground black pepper (for the meat sauce)
- ½ cup mayonnaise as toppings
- 6 oz. shredded cheese as toppings

Instructions:

- We're going to start by cooking the bread. First, preheat the 350 degrees Fahrenheit and then mix all the dry ingredients in a bowl.

- Add some vinegar, egg whites, and boiling water in the bowl. Whisk thoroughly for 30 seconds or use a hand mixer to speed up the process. You'd want a consistency that's a lot like play-doh

- Form the dough into 5 or 8 pieces of bread. Layer then on the lowest oven rack and cook for 55 to 60 minutes.

- In the meantime, you'll be cooking the meat sauce. Grab a pan and cook the onion and garlic until you get that fragrant smell.

- Add the ground beef and cook the meat thoroughly. Once done, add the other ingredients and cook

- Allow it to simmer for 10 minutes in low heat. Add other seasonings to taste.

Nutrition Facts: per serving, you'd get around 57g of protein, 1070 kcalories, 83g fat, 12g fiber, and 15g net carbohydrates

Low Carb Crack Slaw Egg Roll in a Bowl Recipe

Cooking Time: 15 minutes

Servings:

Ingredient List:

- 1 lb. ground beef
- 4 cups shredded coleslaw mix
- 1 tbsp. avocado oil
- 1 tsp. sea salt
- ¼ tsp. black pepper
- 4 cloves garlic, minced
- 3 tbsp. fresh ginger, grated
- ¼ cup coconut aminos
- 2 tsp. toasted sesame oil
- ¼ cup green onions

Instructions:

1. Start by heating the avocado oil in a large pan using a medium-high heat. Put in the garlic and cook for a little bit until you get that fragrant smell.
2. Add the ground beef and cook until it gets brownish. This should take about 10 minutes to finish. Season with salt and black pepper.
3. Once cooked, you can lower the heat and add the coleslaw mix and the coconut aminos. Stir to cook for 5 minutes or until the coleslaw gets tender.

4. Remove and put in the green onions and the toasted sesame oil.

Nutrition Facts: 457 kcalories for 1.5 cups of the dish. Contains 7g carbohydrates, 33g protein, 2g fiber, 2g sugar, and 33g protein.

Low Carb Beef Stir Fry

Cooking Time: 20 minutes

Servings: 2 servings

Ingredient List:

- ½ cup zucchini, spiral them into noodles about 6-inches each
- ¼ cup organic broccoli florets
- 1 bunch baby bok choy, stem chopped
- 2 tbsp. avocado oil
- 2 tsp. coconut aminos
- 1 small know of ginger, peeled and cut
- 8 oz. skirt steak, thinly sliced into strips

Instructions:

1. Heat the pan and add 1 tablespoon of oil. Sear the steak on it on high heat. This should only take around 2 minutes per side.

2. Reduce the heat to medium and put in the broccoli, ginger, ghee, and coconut aminos. Cook for a minute, stirring as often as possible.

3. Add in the bok choy and cook for another minute

4. Finally, put the zucchini into the mix and cook. Note that zucchini noodles cook quickly so you'd want to pay close attention to this.

Nutrition Facts: contains 582 calories, 55g protein, 2g fiber, 36g fat, and 14g carbohydrates.

One Pan Pesto Chicken and Veggies

Cooking Time: 30 minutes

Servings: 4 servings

Ingredient List:

- 2 tbsp. olive oil
- 1 cup cherry diced tomatoes
- ¼ cup basil pesto
- 1/3 cup sun-dried tomatoes, chopped and drained
- 1 pound chicken thigh, bones and skinless, sliced into strips
- 1 pound asparagus, cut in half with the ends trimmed

Instructions:

1. Start by heating up a large skillet. Put two tablespoons of olive oil and sliced chicken on medium heat. Season with salt and add ½ cup of the sun-dried tomatoes.
2. Cook for a few minutes until the chicken is cooked thoroughly. Spoon out the chicken and tomatoes and put them in a separate container.
3. Don't wash the skillet just yet. You'll be using the oil there later.
4. Next, put the asparagus in the skillet and pour in the pesto. Turn the heat on medium and add the remaining sun-dried tomatoes. Cook the asparagus for 5 to 10 minutes. Put it on a separate plate when done.
5. Put the chicken back in the skillet and pour in pesto. Stir under medium heat for 2 minutes. You only need to reheat the chicken during this so when done, you can serve it together with the asparagus.

Nutrition Facts: 423 kcalories, 32g fat, 112mg cholesterol, 261mg sodium, 12g total carbohydrates, and 856mg potassium

Crispy Peanut Tofu and Cauliflower Rice Stir-Fry

Cooking Time: 1 hour and 30 minutes

Servings: 2 servings

Ingredient List:

- 12 oz. tofu, extra-firm
- 1 tbsp. toasted sesame oil
- 2 cloves minced garlic
- 1 small cauliflower head
- 1 ½ tbsp. toasted sesame oil (sauce)
- ½ tsp. chili garlic sauce (sauce)
- 2 ½ tbsp. peanut butter (sauce)
- ¼ cup low sodium soy sauce (sauce)
- ½ cup light brown sugar (sauce)

Instructions:

1. Start by draining the tofu for 90 minutes before getting the meal ready. You can dry the tofu quickly by rolling it on an absorbent towel and putting something heavy on top. This will create a gentle pressure on the tofu to drain out the water.
2. Preheat the oven to 400 degrees Fahrenheit. While the oven heats up, cube the tofu and prepare your baking sheet.
3. Bake for 25 minutes and allow it to cool.
4. Combine the sauce ingredients and whisk it thoroughly until you get that well-blended texture. You can add more ingredients, depending on your personal preferences with taste.

5. Put the tofu in the sauce and stir it quickly to coat the tofu thoroughly. Leave it there for 15 minutes or more for a thorough marinate.

6. While the tofu marinates, shred the cauliflower into rice- size bits. You can also try buying cauliflower rice from the store to save yourself this step. If you're doing this manually, use a fine grater or a food processor.

7. Grab a skillet and put it on medium heat. Start cooking the veggies on a bit of sesame oil and just a little bit of soy sauce. Set it aside.

8. Grab the tofu and put it on the pan. Stir the tofu frequently until it gets that nice golden brown color. Don't worry if some of the tofu sticks to the pan – it will do that sometimes. Set aside.

9. Steam your cauliflower rice for 5 to 8 minutes. Add some sauce and stir thoroughly.

10. Now it's time to add up the ingredients together. Put the cauliflower rice with the veggies and tofu. Serve and enjoy. You can reheat this if there are leftovers, but try not to leave it in the fridge for long.

Nutrition Facts: each serving will have around 524 calories, 34g of fat, 38.5g of carbohydrates, 7g of fiber, 24.5g of protein and 1400mg of sodium

Simple Keto Fried Chicken

Cooking Time: 30 minutes

Servings: 4 servings

Ingredient List:

- 4 boneless and skinless chicken thighs
- Frying oil
- 2 large eggs
- 2 tbsp. heavy whipping cream
- 2/3 cup grated parmesan cheese (breading)
- 2/3 cup blanched almond flour (breading)
- 1 tsp. salt (breading)
- ½ tsp. black pepper (breading)
- ½ tsp. cayenne (breading)
- ½ tsp. paprika (breading)

Instructions:

1. Grab a bowl and put together the eggs and heavy cream. Beat them together until perfectly mixed.
2. Grab another bowl, this time combining all the breading ingredients and mix well. Set it aside for now.
3. Cut the chicken thigh into 3 even pieces. Make sure they're not wet by patting the moist area with a paper towel. This will help prevent the oil splashes when you start frying them.

4. So now you have the chicken and 2 bowls. One bowl contains the egg wash and the other contains the breading. Dip the chicken in the bread first before dipping it in the egg wash and then finally, dipping it in the breading again. Make sure it's completely covered.

5. Put 2 inches worth of oil in a pot and heat it up until it reaches around 350 degrees Fahrenheit or when it starts to become steamy. When this happens, try to gradually lower the heat so you can maintain that temperature. This is important since a perfectly heated oil will help create really crunchy chicken.

6. Put the coated chicken in your hot oil. Do this gently with a pair of tongs, making sure there are no splashes of any kind. Frying time should take around 5 minutes or until the coating becomes deep brown in color.

7. Prepare some paper towels and put the cooked chicken on it. This will help remove any excess oil.

8. Try not to overcrowd the pan so all of them will cook beautifully. Serve while still crispy for best results.

*Nutrition Facts:*380 calories, 2.5g net carbs per serving, 26g of fat, 920mg of sodium, 218mg of cholesterol, 5g total carbohydrates, and 34g of protein.

Keto Butter Chicken

Cooking Time: 30 minutes

Servings: 2 to 4 servings

Ingredient List:

- 1.5 lb. chicken breast
- 1 tbsp. coconut oil
- 2 tbsp. garam masala
- 3 tsp. grated fresh ginger
- 3 tsp. minced garlic
- 4 oz. plain yogurt
- 2 tbsp. butter (for sauce)
- 1 tbsp. ground coriander (for sauce)
- ½ cup heavy cream (for sauce)
- ½ tbsp. garam masala (for sauce)
- 2 tsp. fresh ginger, grated (for sauce)
- 2 tsp. minced garlic (for sauce)
- 2 tsp. cumin (for sauce)
- 1 tsp. chili powder (for sauce)
- 1 onion (for sauce)
- 14.5 oz. crushed tomatoes (for sauce)
- Salt to taste (for sauce)

Instructions:

1. Start by cutting the chicken into pieces measuring around 2 inches each. Place it in a large bowl and add

2 tablespoons of garam masala, 1 teaspoon of minced garlic, and 1 teaspoon of grated ginger. Stir slowly and add the yogurt. Make sure that mix is evenly distributed before putting a lid on the container and chilling it in the fridge for 30 minutes.

2. For the sauce, grab a blender and put in the ginger, garlic, onion, tomatoes, and spices. Blend until smooth.

3. Leave the blended sauce aside and grab a skillet. Using medium heat, remove the chicken from the fridge and cook, allowing it to brown on both sides.

4. Once cooked, pour in the sauce and allow it to simmer for 5 more minutes

5. Finally, put in the cream and ghee, still using medium heat. Add some salt for taste and serve!

Nutrition Facts: contains around 293 calories, 17g of fat, 7g net carbs, and 6g of protein.

Keto Shrimp Scampi Recipe

Cooking Time: 30 minutes

Servings: 2 servings

Ingredient List:

- 2 summer squash

- 1 pound shrimp, deveined
- 2 tbsp. butter unsalted
- 2 tbsp. lemon juice
- 2 tbsp. chopped parsley
- ¼ cup chicken broth
- 1/8 tsp. red chili flakes
- 1 clove minced garlic
- Salt and pepper to taste

Instructions:

- Start by cutting the summer squash into noodle-like shapes. You can use a spiralizer to get this done or perhaps use a fork to scrap the surface.
- Spread the noodles on top of paper towards and sprinkle them with salt. Set aside for 30 minutes.
- Blot the excess water with a paper towel.
- In a frying pan, melt butter over medium heat and fry the garlic until you get that fragrant smell. Add some chicken broth, red chili flakes, and lemon juice.
- Once it boils, add the shrimp and allow it to cook. Reduce the heat once the shrimp turns pink.
- Add more salt and pepper to taste before adding the summer squash noodles and parsley to the mix. Make sure all the ingredients are well-coated by the sauce. Serve.

*Nutrition Facts:*332 kcalories, 8.49g carbohydrates, 48.4g protein, 13.1g fat, 352mg of sodium, 2.3g of fiber, and 187mg of calcium.

Keto Lasagna

Cooking Time: 1 hour and 30 minutes

Servings: 8 servings

Ingredient List:

- 8 oz. block of cream cheese
- 3 large eggs
- Kosher salt
- Ground black pepper
- 2 cups of shredded mozzarella
- ½ cup of freshly grated parmesan
- Pinch crushed red pepper flakes
- Chopped parsley for garnish
- ¾ cup marinara (for the sauce)
- 1 tbsp. tomato paste (for the sauce)
- 1 lb. ground beef (for the sauce)
- ½ cup of freshly grated parmesan (for the sauce)
- 1.5 cup of shredded mozzarella (for the sauce)
- 1 tbsp. of extra virgin olive oil (for the sauce)

- 1 tsp. dried oregano (for the sauce)
- 3 cloves minced garlic (for the sauce)
- ½ cup chopped onion (for the sauce)
- 16 oz. ricotta (for the sauce)

Instructions:

1. Start by preheating the oven to 350 degrees and preparing the baking tray by lining it with parchment and cooking spray.

2. Grab a microwave-safe bowl and throw in the cream cheese, mozzarella, and parmesan, melting them together for a few seconds in the microwave. Mix them in thoroughly before adding the eggs and blending the whole thing together. Add a pinch of salt and pepper for seasoning.

3. Spread the mixture on a baking sheet and bake for 15 to 20 minutes.

4. While baking, grab a skillet and using medium heat, coat the surface with oil. Put in the onion and allow them to cook for 5 minutes before adding the garlic. Once you get that fragrant smell, wait 60 more seconds before adding the tomato paste onto the mixture. Make sure to stir all the items around until the onion and garlic are well-coated.

5. Add the ground beef in the skillet and cook the mixture, breaking up the meat until it's no longer

pink in appearance. Add salt and pepper to taste. Cook it for a few more minutes before setting it aside and allowing it to cool. There should be a bit of fluid remaining in the skillet – try to drain that out of the meat before proceeding with the next step.

6. Turn on the stove again, keeping the medium heat constant. Add some marinara sauce and season with pepper, red pepper flakes, and ground pepper. Stir around to evenly distribute the flavor.

7. By this time, your noodles should be ready from the oven. Take them out and start cutting them in half width-wise and then cut them again into 3 pieces.

8. Start layering! Use an 8 inch baking pan for this, placing 2 noodles at the bottom of the dish first and layer as you wish. Alternate the parmesan and mozzarella shreds depending on your personal preferences.

9. Bake until the cheese melts and the sauce bubbles out. Should take about 30 minutes.

10. Garnish and serve.

*Nutrition Facts:*308 calories, 21.7 grams of fat, 852 grams of sodium, 0.5 grams of dietary fiber, 2.2 grams of carbohydrates, and 23.3 grams of protein.

Creamy Tuscan Garlic Chicken

Cooking Time: 20 to 25 minutes

Servings: 6 servings

Ingredient List:

- 1.5 pounds boneless and skinless chicken breast, thinly sliced
- ½ cup chicken broth
- ½ cup parmesan cheese
- ½ cup sun dried tomatoes
- 1 cup heavy cream
- 1 cup chopped spinach
- 2 tbsp. olive oil
- 1 tsp. garlic powder
- 1 tsp. Italian seasoning

Instructions:

1. Grab a large skillet and cook the chicken using olive oil using medium heat. Do this for 5 minutes for each side or until they're thoroughly cooked. Set it aside in a plate.
2. Using the same skillet, combine the heavy cream, garlic powder, Italian seasoning, parmesan cheese, and chicken broth. Expose it to medium heat and just whisk away until the mixture thickens.

3. Add the sundried tomatoes and spinach and let it simmer until the spinach wilts.
4. Add the chicken back and serve.

Nutrition Facts: per serving, you have 368 calories from fat which amounts to 25 grams of fat, 133 mg of cholesterol, 379mg of sodium, 7g of carbohydrates, 1g of fiber, 4g sugar, and 30g protein.

Keto Snack Recipes

Parmesan Cheese Strips

Cooking Time: 30 minutes

Servings: 12 servings

Ingredient List:

- 1 cup shredded parmesan cheese
- 1 tsp dried basil

Instructions:

1. Preheat the oven to 350 degrees Fahrenheit. Prepare the baking sheet by lining it with parchment paper.
2. Form small piles of the parmesan cheese on the baking sheet. Flatten it out evenly and then sprinkle dried basil on top of the cheese.

3. Bake for 5 to 7 minutes or until you get a gold brown color with crispy edges. Take it out, serve, and enjoy!

Nutrition Facts: contains 31 calories, 2g fat, and 2g protein

Peanut Butter Power Granola

Cooking Time: 40 minutes

Servings: 12 servings

Ingredient List:

- 1 cup shredded coconut or almond flour
- 1 1/2 cups almonds
- 1 1/2 cups pecans
- 1/3 cup swerve sweetener
- 1/3 cup vanilla whey protein powder
- 1/3 cup peanut butter
- 1/4 cup sunflower seeds
- 1/4 cup butter
- 1/4 cup water

Instructions:

1. Preheat the oven to 300 degrees Fahrenheit and prepare a baking sheet with parchment paper
2. Place the almonds and pecans in a food processor. Put them all in a large bowl and add the sunflower

seeds, shredded coconut, vanilla, sweetener, and protein powder.

3. Melt the peanut butter and butter together in the microwave.

4. Mix the melted butter in the nut mixture and stir it thoroughly until the nuts are well-distributed.

5. Put in the water to create a lumpy mixture.

6. Scoop out small amounts of the mixture and place it on the baking sheet.

7. Bake for 30 minutes. Enjoy!

Nutrition Facts: 338kcalories, 30g fat, 5g carbohydrates, 9.6g protein, and 5g fiber

Homemade Graham Crackers

Cooking Time: 1 hour 10 minutes

Servings: 10 servings

Ingredient List:

- 1 egg, large
- 2 cups almond flour
- 1/3 cup swerve brown
- 2 tsp cinnamon
- 1 tsp baking powder
- 2 tbsp melted butter

- 1 tsp vanilla extract
- salt

Instructions:

1. Preheat the oven to 300 degrees Fahrenheit
2. Grab a bowl and whisk the almond flour, cinnamon, sweetener, baking powder, and salt. Stir all the ingredients together.
3. Put in the egg, molasses, melted butter, and vanilla extract. Stir until you get a dough-like consistency.
4. Roll out the dough evenly, making sure that you don't go beyond ¼ of an inch thick. Cut the dough into the shapes you want for cooking. Transfer it on the baking tray
5. Bake for 20 to 30 minutes until it firms up. Let it cool for 30 minutes outside of the oven and then put them back in for another 30 minutes. Make sure that for the second time putting the biscuit, the temperature is not higher than 200 degrees Fahrenheit. This last step will make the biscuit crispy.

Nutrition Facts: 156 kcalories, 13.35g fat, 6.21g carbohydrates, 5.21g protein, and 2.68g fiber.

Keto No Bake Cookies

Cooking Time: 10 minutes

Servings: 18 cook

Ingredient List:

- 2/3 cup of all natural peanut butter
- 1 cup of all natural shredded coconut, unsweetened
- 2 tbsp real butter
- 4 drops of vanilla lakanto

Instructions:

1. Melt the butter in the microwave.
2. Take it out and put in the peanut butter. Stir thoroughly.
3. Add the sweetener and coconut. Mix.
4. Spoon it onto a pan lined with parchment paper
5. Freeze for 10 minutes
6. Cut into preferred slices. Store in an airtight container in the fridge and enjoy whenever.

Nutrition Facts: 80 calories per serving.

Swiss Cheese Crunchy Nachos

Cooking Time: 20 minutes

Servings: 2 servings

Ingredient List:

- ½ cup shredded Swiss cheese
- ½ cup shredded cheddar cheese
- 1/8 cup cooked bacon pieces

Instructions:

- Preheat the oven to 300 degrees Fahrenheit and prepare the baking sheet by lining it with parchment paper.
- Start by spreading the Swiss cheese on the parchment. Sprinkle it with bacon and then top it off again with the cheese.
- Bake until the cheese has melted. This should take around 10 minutes or less.
- Allow the cheese to cool before cutting them into triangle strips.
- Grab another baking sheet and place the triangle cheese strips on top. Broil them for 2 to 3 minutes so they'll get chunky.

Nutrition Facts: 280 calories per serving, 21.8 fat, 18.6g protein, and 2.44g net carbohydrates

Homemade Thin Mints

Cooking Time: 60 minutes

Servings: 20 servings

Ingredient List:

- 1 egg slightly beaten
- 1 3/4 cups almond flour
- 1/3 cup cocoa powder
- 1/3 cup swerve sweetener
- 2 tbsp butter melted
- 1 tsp baking powder
- 1/2 tsp vanilla extract
- 1/4 tsp salt
- 1 tbsp coconut oil (coating)
- 7 oz sugar free dark chocolate (coating)
- 1 tsp peppermint extract (coating)

Instructions:

1. Preheat the oven to 300 degrees Fahrenheit. Prepare the baking sheet by lining it with parchment paper.
2. Grab a large bowl and combine the cacao powder, sweetener, almond flour, salt, and baking powder. Mix thoroughly before adding the already beaten egg, vanilla extract and butter.
3. Knead the dough and roll it on the parchment paper. Make sure it doesn't go beyond a thickness of ¼ inch.

4. Cut the cookie into your desired shapes. Combine and reroll, cut it up and again and repeat until nothing is left.

5. Bake the cookies for 20 to 30 minutes.

6. For the coating, melt the oil and chocolate in a bowl and stir until it's completely smooth. Use a microwave to do this or make sure of a pan placed in boiling water.

7. Once melted, stir in the peppermint extract.

8. Take the cookies and dip them in the coating, depending on your personal preferences. Allow it to dry on the surface and then refrigerate to keep it fresh.

Nutrition Facts: 116kcalories per 2 calories, 10.41g fat, 6.99g carbohydrates, 8g protein, 5mg cholesterol

Mozzarella Cheese Pockets

Cooking Time:

Servings: 8 servings

Ingredient List:

- 1 large egg
- 8 pcs of mozzarella cheese sticks, whole
- 1 ¾ cup mozzarella cheese

- ¾ cup almond flour
- 1 oz. cream cheese
- ½ cup of crushed pork rinds

Instructions:

1. Start by grating the mozzarella cheese.
2. In a bowl, mix together the almond flour, mozzarella, and the cream cheese. Microwave them for 30 seconds until you get that delicious gooey mixture.
3. Put in a large egg and mix the whole thing together. You should get a nice thick batch of dough.
4. Put the dough in between two wax papers and roll it around until you get a semi-rectangular shape
5. Cut them into smaller rectangle pieces and wrap them around the cheese sticks. Mold it depending on the shape you want.
6. Roll the stick onto crushed pork rinds.
7. Bake for 20 to 25 minutes at 400 degrees Fahrenheit. You can also try deep frying them if you have Keto-friendly oil options.
8. You can store them in the fridge if you don't want to cook them just yet. When serving, try using Keto-friendly ketchup or just some marinara sauce.

*Nutrition Facts:*272 calories, 22g fat, 2.4g net carbohydrates, and 17g protein. Note that the dipping you use is a different nutrition count.

No Bake Coconut Cookies

Cooking Time: 10 minutes

Servings: 8 servings

Ingredient List:

- 3 cups of unsweetened shredded coconut
- ½ cup sweetener
- 3/8 cup coconut oil
- 3/8 tsp. salt or to taste
- 2 tsp. vanilla
- Optional toppings: coconut shreds or finely-chopped nuts

Instructions:

1. Put all the ingredients in a food processor without the optional toppings. You can also use the blender but try not to turn it too high because you'll end with a liquefied mix which won't produce the cookies in this recipe.
2. Remove and start forming them into the shape you want. Decorate as you want with the toppings.
3. Leave them to firm up for as long as necessary. This shouldn't take more than a few hours.
4. Store in the fridge to lengthen its shelf life.

*Nutrition Facts:*329 kcalories, 4.1g carbohydrates, 2.1g protein, 30g fat, 122mg sodium, 2.3g sugar, 25.7g saturated fat, and .39g polyunsaturated fat.

Cheesy Cauliflower Breadsticks

Cooking Time: 45 minutes to1 hour

Servings: each serving should be around 99 grams

Ingredient List:

- 4 eggs
- 4 cups of cauliflower riced
- 2 cups mozzarella cheese
- 4 cloves minced garlic
- 3 tsp. oregano
- Salt and pepper to taste

Instructions:

1. Start by preheating your oven to 425 degrees Fahrenheit.
2. Prepare the baking sheet by lining it with parchment paper.
3. Put cauliflower in a food processor or blender until finely chopped or when it resembles rice.

4. Put it in a covered bowl and microwave for just 10 minutes. Allow it to cool and if it's a little wet, make sure to drain it first before adding eggs, oregano, garlic, salt, pepper, and mozzarella. Mix them well.

5. Start separating the mixture into individual sticks – or really, just about any form you want.

6. Bake the crust for 25 minutes or until it gets that nice golden color. Take it out of the oven and sprinkle some more mozzarella on top while still hot. Put it back in the oven for just 5 minutes so that the cheese melts.

7. Bonus! You can also use the same recipe as a pizza crust.

Nutrition Facts: each 99 gram stick contains kcalories, 4 grams carbohydrates, 13 grams protein, 11 grams fat, 114 mg cholesterol, 310 mg sodium, 1 gram fiber, 232 mg potassium, and 1 gram sugar.

Easy Peanut Butter Cups

Cooking Time: 1 hour 35 minutes

Servings: 12 servings

Ingredient List:

- 1/2 cup peanut butter

- 1/4 cup butter
- 3 oz. cacao butter, chopped
- 1/3 cup powdered swerve sweetener
- 1/2 tsp vanilla extract
- 4 oz. sugar free dark chocolate

Instructions:

1. Line a muffin tin with parchment paper or cupcake liners.
2. Using low heat, melt the peanut butter, butter, and cacao butter in a saucepan. Stir them until completely combined.
3. Add the vanilla and sweetener until there are no more lumps.
4. Carefully place the mixture in the muffin cups.
5. Refrigerate it until firm
6. Put chocolate in a bowl and set the bowl in boiling water. This is done to avoid direct contact with the heat. Stir the chocolate until completely melted.
7. Take the muffin out of the fridge and drizzle in the chocolate on top. Put it back again in the fridge to firm it up. This should take 15 minutes to finish.
8. Store and serve when needed.

Nutrition Facts: 200kcalories, 19g fat, 6g carbohydrates, 2.9g protein and 3.6g fiber

Keto Dessert Recipes

Keto Cheesecake with Blueberries

Cooking Time: 1 hour 30 minutes

Servings: 12 servings

Ingredient List:

- 1¼ cups almond flour (crust)
- 2 tbsp erythritol (crust)
- ½ tsp of vanilla extract (crust)
- 2 oz. butter (crust)
- 20 oz. cream cheese (filling)
- 2 eggs (filling)
- 1 egg yolk (filling)
- ½ cup of crème fraîche or heavy whipping cream (filling)
- 1 tsp lemon zest (filling)
- ½ tsp of vanilla extract (filling)
- 2 oz. fresh blueberries (optional)

Instructions:

1. Preheat the oven to 350 degrees Fahrenheit. While waiting, prepare a springform pan by lining it with butter or putting in parchment paper.

2. Melt the butter until you smell that nutty scent. This will help create a toffee flavor for the crust.
3. Remove the pan from the heat and add almond flour, vanilla, and the sweetener. Mix the ingredients until you get a dough-like consistency.
4. Press it into the pan and bake for 8 minutes until you get a slightly golden crust. Set aside to cool.
5. Now we're going to work on the filling. Mix all the filling ingredients together and beat it heavily. Pour the mixture on the crust.
6. Increase the oven's heat to 400 degrees Fahrenheit and bake for the next 15 minutes
7. Once done, lower it to 230 degrees Fahrenheit and bake again for 45 to 60 minutes
8. Turn the heat off and leave it inside in the oven to cool.
9. Remove after it has cooled completely. You can store it in the fridge and served with fresh blueberries on top.

Nutrition Facts: each slice contains 4g net carbohydrates, 33g fat, 7g protein, and 335 kcalories

Keto Lemon Ice Cream

Cooking Time: 1 hour 30 minutes

123

Servings: 6 servings

Ingredient List:

- 3 eggs
- 1 lemon, zest and juice
- ⅓ cup erythritol
- 1¾ cups heavy whipping cream

Instructions:

1. Grate the lemon to get the zest and then squeeze out the juice. Set it aside in the meantime.
2. Separate the eggs. Using a hand mixer beat the eggs until they become stiff. Afterwards, beat the egg yolks and sweetener until it becomes light and fluffy.
3. Add the lemon juice in the egg yolks. Beat it before carefully folding the egg whites into the yolk.
4. In a separate bowl, whip the cream until you get soft peak. Gently fold the egg mix into the cream
5. Pour the whole thing into an ice cream maker and use it according to instructions of the manufacturer.
6. For those who don't have an ice cream maker, you can just put the bowl in the freezer. You'll have to take it out every 30 minutes to stir it. This should be done for the next two hours until you get the consistency you want.

Nutrition Facts: contains 27g fat, 5g protein, 3g net carbohydrates, and 269 kcalories

Peanut Butter Balls

Cooking Time: 20 minutes

Servings: 18 servings

Ingredient List:

- 1 cup of salted peanuts chopped finely (not peanut flour)
- 1 cup of peanut butter
- 1 cup of sweetener
- 8 oz of sugar free chocolate chips

Instructions:

1. Mix the peanut butter, sweetener, and chopped peanuts together. You'll get a dough-light substance by doing this.
2. Knead until smooth and then divide the dough into 18 pieces. Shape them into balls.
3. Place the dough on a baking sheet lined with wax paper before putting them in the fridge to harden.
4. In the meantime, melt the chocolate chips in a microwave.
5. Take out the peanut butter balls and dip them in the melted chocolate. Put them back in the fridge to set. Enjoy!

Nutrition Facts: 194 kcalories, 17g total fat, 7g carbohydrates, 1g sugar, and 7g protein.

Keto Cake Donuts

Cooking Time: 30 minutes

Servings: 8 servings

Ingredient List:

- 6 eggs
- ½ cup coconut flour
- ¼ tsp sea salt
- ¼ tsp baking soda
- 1 tsp vanilla extract
- ¼ tsp almond extract
- ½ cup butter or coconut oil
- ½ cup erythritol
- ½ tsp of vanilla extract (frosting)
- ¼ cup melted butter or coconut oil (frosting)
- ¼ cup cream cheese, softened (frosting)
- ¼ cup powdered erythritol (frosting)
- 3 tbsp melted butter (chocolate drizzle)
- 2 tbsp powdered erythritol (chocolate drizzle)
- 1 tbsp cocoa powder, unsweetened (chocolate drizzle)

Instructions:

1. Start by preheating the oven to 350 degrees Celsius Fahrenheit
2. Grab a large bowl and out in the donut ingredients.

3. Take a greased donut pan and will it with batter around 2/3 of the way

4. Bake for 20 minutes.

5. While waiting, start making the frosting. Do this by putting all the frosting ingredients in a bowl and stir completely with a hand mixer. Add sugar to taste.

6. Dip the now cool donuts in the frosting and set it on the parchment to cool.

7. For the chocolate drizzle, put all the ingredients in a small bowl and stir. Drizzle with the liquid as desired.

Nutrition Facts: contains 294 kcalories, 2g net carbohydrates 4g fiber, 28g fat, and 6g protein

Chocolate Coconut Candies

Cooking Time: 20 minutes

Servings: 20 mini cups

Ingredient List:

- 1/2 cup coconut butter
- 1/2 cup Kelapo coconut oil
- 1/2 cup unsweetened shredded coconut
- 3 tbsp powdered swerve sweetener powdered swerve sweeter
- 1 ½ oz. cocoa butter (topping)

- 1 oz. unsweetened chocolate (topping)
- ½ cup cocoa powder (topping)
- 1/4 cup powdered swerve sweetener (topping)
- 4 tsp vanilla extract (topping)

Instructions:

1. Start by lining the mini muffin with paper liners.
2. Put the coconut oil and coconut butter in a saucepan and melt it using low heat. Stir completely before adding the shredded coconut and sweetener into the mix.
3. Divide the mixture onto the mini muffin cups. Set them aside so they'll become firm.
4. In a separate pan, put cocoa butter and unsweetened chocolate together. Melt them by setting the container in a pan of boiling water. This is done to avoid directly heat on the pan containing the chocolate.
5. Put the powdered sweetener and cocoa powder slowly until it smoothens into a thick consistency.
6. Remove it from the heat and put the vanilla extract. Blend carefully.
7. Spoon the chocolate topping on the firm coconut candies. Wait 15 to 20 minutes for it to set.

Nutrition Facts: 240kcalories, 5g carbohydrates, 4g of fiber, 25g fat, 2g protein, 6mg sodium

Flourless Chocolate Cake

Cooking Time: 1 hour

Servings: 12 servings

Ingredient List:

- 4 large eggs
- 1/3 cup water
- 1/2 sugar substitute
- 12 ounces unsweetened baking chocolate
- 2/3 cup butter or ghee, cut into tablespoon size pieces
- 1/4 teaspoon salt
- Boiling water

Instructions:

1. Start by preparing the springform pan for cooking by lining it with parchment paper.
2. Grab a small pot and apply medium heat. Put in the water, salt, and sweetener until fully dissolved.
3. Using a microwave, melt the baking chocolate.
4. Mix the melted chocolate and the butter using an electric mixer
5. Add it in the hot water mixture and beat thoroughly until well blended.
6. Beat the eggs in a separate container and slowly add into the mixture. Combine it thoroughly

7. Pour the resulting mixture in the pan and wrap the exterior with foil.

8. Now put the pan in a larger cake pan. Put boiling water outside of the pan, keeping the depth at just 1 inch.

9. Bake the cake in the water for 45 minutes at 350 degrees Fahrenheit. Chill it in the fridge overnight before serving.

Nutrition Facts: Contains 295kcalories, 8g carbohydrates, 6g protein, 1g polyunsaturated fat, 16g saturated fat, and 5g fiber.

No Bake Low Carb Lemon Strawberry Cheesecake

Cooking Time: 15 to 20 minutes

Servings: 2 servings

Ingredient List:

- 3 oz. cream cheese, softened
- ¾ cup heavy whipping cream
- 1/3 cup sweetener
- 2 tsps. Lemon extract
- 2 large strawberries, chopped
- Lemon zest

Instructions:

1. Grab a mixing bowl and put in the cream cheese, whipping cream, and sweetener. Beat all three on high until you get that smooth and creamy consistency.

2. Put in the lemon extract and mix again. Grate in the lemon zest if you want that additional lemony flavor, otherwise you won't need it at all.

3. Put the cream cheese mixture into your containers. Sprinkle some of the strawberries in between just to add some layer into the mix. Completely fill your container and then sprinkle some more of the strawberries on top. If you have some more lemon zest, you can sprinkle those on top too.

4. Refrigerate until you're ready to eat.

Nutrition Facts: contains 474 calories, 5.7g carbs, 0.4g fiber, 48.2g fat, and 4.5g protein.

Keto Fudge Recipe

Cooking Time: 1 hour

Servings: 12 servings

Ingredient List:

- 1 cup solid coconut oil
- 1 tsp. vanilla extract

- 1/8 tsp. sea salt
- ¼ cup powdered erythritol, to taste
- ¼ cup cocoa powder

Instructions:

1. Start by lining a rectangular glass container with parchment paper.
2. Keeping it at low speed, use a hand mixer to beat the coconut oil together with the sweetener until fully combined.
3. Add in the cocoa powder, vanilla, and sea salt to taste. Add some of the sweetener according to your personal preferences. Beat further with a hand mixer
4. Transfer the mix to the container. Smoothen out the surface.
5. Refrigerate for 45 to 60 minutes or until fully solid. Sprinkle the top portion with sea salt flakes or any other topping you might want.

Nutrition Facts: 161 kcalories per cube, 18 grams of fat, 0.6 grams fiber.

Low Carbohydrate Brownie

Cooking Time: 3 minutes

Servings: 1 serving

Ingredient List:

- 1 whole egg
- 32 grams or 1 scoop of chocolate protein powder
- 1 tbsp. coconut flour
- 1 tbsp. granulates sweetener (optional)
- 1 tbsp. cocoa powder
- 1 tbsp. chocolate chunks (optional)
- ½ tsp. baking powder
- ¼ cup milk

Instructions:

1. Start by mixing all the dry ingredients first and combining them thoroughly.
2. Add the wet ingredients next until you get a nice and thick batter. The thickness depends on your personal preference so if you think it's too much, you can try adding spoonful's of milk until you're happy with the results.
3. Grease a microwave safe bowl and pour in the resulting mix. Cooking it via the microwave should take around 55 to 60 seconds. Feel free to take it out every now and then until you get the texture you want.
4. Some people use an oven for this. If you do, try cooking at a temperature of 350 degrees Fahrenheit for 12 to 15 minutes.

Nutrition Facts: 100kcalories

Keto Friendly Ice Cream

Cooking Time: 30 to 40 minutes exclusive of the freezing process

Servings: ½ cup

Ingredient List:

- 3 tbsp. butter
- 3 cups heavy cream, separated
- 1/3 cup powdered erythritol
- ¼ cup MCT oil or MCT oil powder
- 1 tsp. vanilla extract
- 1 medium vanilla bean, scraped

Instructions:

- Start by melting the butter over medium heat. Add around 2 cups of heavy cream and erythritol together and allow it to boil before reducing the heat. Let it simmer for the next 30 to 45 minutes. Stir it occasionally to check the consistency of the mixture. There should be an obvious decrease of volume when you heat it up. The cream should thoroughly coat the back of a spoon if you try to take some out.
- Once done, pour the concoction into a large bowl and let it cool. Put in the vanilla extract and vanilla seeds afterwards. Add the MCT oil or oil powder and whisk.

- Pour in the last cup of heavy cream and whisk again until you get the beautiful smooth consistency.
- Now, once you're done with this, you have two options: you can make ice cream with an ice cream maker or you can just use your freezer.
- If you're using an ice cream maker, just churn the mixture according to the instructions of the ice cream maker. Store in the fridge and enjoy!
- If you don't have an ice cream maker, you can still have ice cream! It's important though that you added the MCT oil or oil powder – otherwise you might not get the results you want. To use the freezer, just line the ice cream container with parchment paper and put it all inside. Freeze the whole mix for 5 to 6 hours, making sure to stir the ice cream every 30 minutes during the first 2 hours. After that, you can stir it every 60 minutes.
- Once done, serve!

*Nutrition Facts:*347 kcalories, 36g of fat, 2g protein, 3g total carbohydrates, and 2g of sugar.

Keto Vegan Recipes

Before I start talking about Keto Vegan recipes, it's important to first talk about these two different concepts. Of course, we already talked about the Ketogenic Diet, but what about Veganism? The first thing you should remember is that Vegan is different from Vegetarian. A vegetarian is fairly obvious – it's a diet that refuses animal meat. Veganism however refuses everything produced by animals. Hence, a vegetarian will eat eggs and milk because it's not animal meat. A vegan however will not drink milk or eat eggs because they came from animal, even if you didn't have to kill anything to get them.

So now that we've made that explanation, here are some popular Ketogenic Vegan recipes.

Chocolate Sea Salt Smoothie

Cooking Time: 5 minutes

Servings: 2 servings

Ingredient List:

- 1 avocado (frozen or not)
- 2 cups almond milk
- 1 tbsp tahini
- ¼ cup cocoa powder
- 1 scoop perfect Keto chocolate base

Instructions:

1. Combine all the ingredients in a high speed blender and mix until you get a soft smoothie.
2. Add ice and enjoy!

Nutrition Facts: contains 235 calories, 20g fat, 11.25 carbohydrates, 8g fiber, and 5.5g protein

8 Ingredient Zucchini Lasagna

Cooking Time: 1 hour 20 minutes

Servings: 9 servings

Ingredient List:

- 3 cups raw macadamia nuts or soaked blanched almonds (for ricotta)
- 2 tbsp nutritional yeast (for ricotta)
- 2 tsp dried oregano (for ricotta)
- 1 tsp sea salt (for ricotta)
- 1/2 cup water or more as needed (for ricotta)
- 1/4 cup vegan parmesan cheese (for ricotta)
- 1/2 cup fresh basil, chopped (for ricotta)
- 1 medium lemon, juiced (for ricotta)
- Black pepper to taste (for ricotta)
- 1 28-oz jar favorite marinara sauce

- 3 medium zucchini squash thinly sliced with a mandolin

Instructions:

1. Preheat the oven to 375 degrees Fahrenheit

2. Put macadamia nuts to a food processor.

3. Add the remaining ingredients and continue to puree the mixture. You want to create a fine paste.

4. Taste and adjust the seasonings depending on your personal preferences.

5. Pour 1 cup of marinara sauce in a baking dish.

6. Start creating the lasagna layers using thinly sliced zucchini

7. Scoop small amounts of ricotta mixture on the zucchini and spread it into a thin layer. Continue the layering until you've run out of zucchini or space for it.

8. Sprinkle parmesan cheese on the topmost layer.

9. Cover the pan with foil and bake for 45 minutes.

10. Remove the foil and bake for 15 minutes more.

11. Allow it to cool for 15 minutes before serving. Serve immediately.

12. The lasagna will keep for 3 days in the fridge.

Nutrition Facts: Contains 338 calories, 34g fat, 10g carbohydrates, 5g fiber, 4.7g protein.

Vegan Keto Scramble

Cooking Time: 10 to 15 minutes

Servings: 1 serving

Ingredient List:

- 14 oz. firm tofu
- 3 tbsp. avocado oil
- 2 tbsp. yellow onion, diced
- 1.5 tbsp. nutritional yeast
- ½ tsp. turmeric
- ½ tsp. garlic powder
- ½ tsp. salt
- 1 cup baby spinach
- 3 grape tomatoes
- 3 oz. vegan cheddar cheese

Instructions:

1. Start by squeezing the water out of the tofu block using a clean cloth or a paper towel.

2. Grab a skillet and put it on medium heat. Sauté the chopped onion in a small amount of avocado oil until it starts to caramelize

3. Using a potato masher, crumble the tofu on the skillet. Do this thoroughly until the tofu looks a lot like scrambled eggs.

4. Drizzle some more of the avocado oil onto the mix together with the dry seasonings. Stir thoroughly and evenly distribute the flavor.

5. Cook under medium heat, occasionally stirring to avoid burning of the tofu. You'd want most of the liquid to evaporate until you get a nice chunk of scrambled tofu.

6. Fold the baby spinach, cheese, and diced tomato. Cook for a few more minutes until the cheese melted. Serve and enjoy!

*Nutrition Facts:*212 calories, 17.5g of fat, 4.74g of net carbohydrates, and 10g of protein

Keto Soup Recipes

Low Carb Vegetarian Ramen

Cooking Time: 30 minutes

Servings: 4 servings

Ingredient List:

- 4 cups filtered water
- 4 pastured eggs
- 1 tbsp sugar-free red curry paste
- 1 tbsp coconut oil
- 2 tsp ground ginger
- 1 tsp ground turmeric
- 1 tsp garlic powder
- 2 cups full-fat canned coconut milk
- 1 cup of purple cabbage, chopped
- 1 cup of large-sized shredded rainbow carrots
- 1 cup Brussels sprouts, halved
- 2 large zucchinis, spiralized
- Salt and pepper to taste

Instructions:

1. Grab a large pot and pour the water inside it, bringing it to a boil.

2. When boiling, add the coconut milk and spices. Reduce the heat to medium-low.

3. Put in the cabbage, brussel sprouts, and carrots. Stir in a while before adding the curry paste and coconut oil.

4. Cook until the vegetables are soft and tender. This should take about 20 minutes

5.   While waiting, soft boil the eggs. This should take about 6 minutes. Take it out of the pot and put in cold water.

6.   When the vegetables are soft, put in the zucchini and allow it to cook for 4 minutes.

7.   Your vegetarian ramen is ready. Serve it with the peeled and halved eggs.

8.   Put in some lime juice and cilantro.

Nutrition Facts: 237 calories, 15g fat, 15g total carbohydrates, 4g fiber, 7g sugar and 10g protein.

Low Carb Smoked Salmon Chowder

Cooking Time: 20 minutes

Servings: 6 servings

Ingredient List:

- 1 stalk celery chopped
- 1 clove garlic minced
- 2 tbsp salted butter
- 2 tbsp capers
- 2 tbsp chopped red onion
- 1 tbsp tomato paste
- ½ tsp salt

- ¼ cup chopped onion
- 1½ cups chicken broth
- 1½ cups heavy whipping cream
- 4 oz cream cheese
- 6 oz smoked salmon hot smoked, chopped

Instructions:

1.   Grab a large saucepan and melt butter in it using medium heat.

2.   Put onion, celery, and sprinkle some salt onto the pan.

3.   Sauté until the vegetables are tender.

4.   Put in the onion until fragrant.

5.   Add the chicken broth and tomato paste.

6.   Allow the mix to simmer, constantly stirring until you get a smooth concoction.

7.   In the meantime, put the cream cheese in a blender and put some of the broth mixture inside it. Blend until smooth. You can do this slowly if this will make it easier.

8.   Put the broth back in the saucepan and add the salmon, capers, and cream.

9.   Allow it to simmer again for a few minutes. The soup is ready now. Before serving, try sprinkling some chopped red onion on top.

Nutrition Facts: 373 kcalories, 31.84g carbohydrates,0.5g fiber, and 12.9g protein.

Keto Bone Broth

Cooking Time: 24 hours

Servings: 12 servings

Ingredient List:

- 3 Pastured Chicken Carcasses
- 10 cups of filtered water
- 2 tbsp. peppercorns
- 3 tsp turmeric
- 1 tsp salt
- 2 tbsp apple cider vinegar
- 1 lemon
- 3 bay leaves

Instructions:

1. Preheat the oven to 400 degrees Fahrenheit.
2. Put the bones on a sheet pan and slightly sprinkle with salt. Roast the chicken for 45 minutes.
3. Transfer the cooked chicken to the slow cooker bowl. Put in the peppercorns, apple cider vinegar, water, and bay leaves

4.   Cook on low heat for 23 hours.

5.   When done, strain the bowl using a fine mesh sieve.

6.   Discard the solid ingredients.

7.   Divide the broth in mason jars, about 2 cups each container.

8.   Put in 1 tsp of turmeric for each day and 2 slices of lemon.

9.   If you're putting it in a large container, just make sure to maintain the ration. Hence, if the large container has 4 cups worth of broth, you should put 2 teaspoons of turmeric and 4 slices of lemon inside.

10.   Heat slowly and serve when needed

Nutrition Facts: contains 70 calories, 4g of fat, 1g carbohydrates, and 6g protein

Note: This is a base recipe, which means you can use it for making other soup recipes provided in this Chapter. Feel free to alter it slightly, depending on your personal preferences.

Slow Cooker Vegetable Beef Soup

Cooking Time: 6 hours 30 minutes

Servings: 12 servings

Ingredient List:

- 4 slices bacon sliced into 1/2 inch pieces
- 2 pounds stew meat cut into 1" cubes, patted dry
- 1 small celeriac diced
- 2 tbsp red wine vinegar
- 2 tbsp tomato paste
- 1/2 tsp dried rosemary
- 1/2 tsp dried thyme
- 1/2 tsp ground black pepper
- 1 tsp sea salt
- 1/4 cup green beans cut into 1 inch pieces
- 1/4 cup carrots diced
- 1 28 oz can diced tomatoes
- 2 cloves garlic crushed
- 32 oz beef broth low-sodium
- 1 medium yellow onion chopped

Instructions:

1.   Put a large skillet on medium high heat. Cook bacon until crispy and store it in the fridge for later.

2.   Remove most of the bacon grease, keeping only a small amount enough to cook the beef cubes in small batches. Season them with salt and pepper.

3.   Cook until the beef cubes are browned. You don't have to cook the meat thoroughly, just sear it a little at the side.

4.   When brown, place the beef in a slow cooker crock.

5.   Once all the beef cubes are in the slow cooker, turn your attention to the skillet. Lower the heat to medium and add vinegar to the skillet.

6.   Stir the vinegar around until you get a thicker consistency.

7.   Pour ¼ cup of the broth in the skillet.

8.   When done, pour the liquid in the slow cooker.

9.   Remember, we only transferred ¼ cup of the broth to the skillet. The remaining broth will now be cooked in the pan. This time, you'll beading the celeriac, carrots, diced tomatoes, tomato paste, onion, green beans, rosemary, thyme, and salt to the mixture. Put some pepper as well depending on the taste.

10.   Cook for 5 minutes before transferring the whole thin to the slow cooker as well.

11.   Stir constantly for 5 minutes.

12.   Cover the slow cooker and set it to run for 7 hours. Taste every 2 hours and adjust as needed. Garnish with the bacon bits when serving.

Nutrition Facts: contains 212 calories per serving, 13g of fat, 6g of carbohydrates, 1g of fiber, 17g of protein, and 5g of net carbohydrates.

Beef Cabbage Soup

Cooking Time: 35 minutes

Servings: 8 people

Ingredient List:

- 1 pound scotch fillet steak, cut into 1-inch pieces
- 1 large onion, chopped
- 1 stalk celery, chopped
- 2 large carrots, diced
- 1 small green cabbage chopped into bite-sized pieces
- 4 cloves garlic minced
- 6 cups beef stock or broth
- 3 tbsp fresh chopped parsley plus more to serve
- 2 tbsp olive oil
- 2 tsp dried thyme
- 2 tsp dried rosemary
- 2 tsp onion or garlic powder
- Salt and freshly-cracked black pepper to taste

Instructions:

1. Put oil in a large pot and apply medium heat.
2. Sear the beef on all sides until brown. They don't have to be cooked as they will be cooked later.

3.   Put in the onions and cook them for 3 minutes

4.   Put the celery and carrots. Cook them while constantly stirring for 4 minutes

5.   Put in the cabbage and continue cooking until the cabbage softens up. Put in the garlic until you get that very fragrant flavor.

6.   Add the stock or broth. Follow it up with the dried herbs, parsley, and the onion or garlic powder. Remember that you're using low to medium heat all this time.

7.   Mix well and bring it to a simmer. Cover the pot with a lid and leave it like that for 15 minutes.

8.   Constantly check to see if the carrots are already cooked as these will take the longest. When they're already soft, season the soup with salt and pepper to taste.

9.   Serve hot and enjoy! You can keep this in the fridge for up to 3 days or even 2 months if you freeze them.

Nutrition Facts: contains 177kcalories per serving, 4g carbohydrates, 12g protein, 11g fat, 2g sugar, and 34mg cholesterol

Keto Chicken Soup

Cooking Time: 40 minutes

Servings: 4 servings

Ingredient List:

- 2 tbsp avocado oil
- 2 stalks celery, chopped
- 4 cups chicken broth
- 2 cups riced cauliflower
- 1/2 tsp dried thyme leaves
- 1/2 tsp paprika
- 1/4 cup chopped onions
- 2 cloves garlic, minced
- 1 lb of skinless, boneless chicken thighs, cubed
- salt & pepper, to taste

Instructions:

1. Start by grabbing a large saucepan and heating the oil over medium heat.
2. Put in the onion and celery. Season it with salt and pepper before cooking.
3. Wait until the vegetable becomes soft before adding the garlic, paprika, and thyme. You should be able to get a fragrant smell
4. Put in the broth and stir for a few minutes.

5.   Add the riced cauliflower and the chicken. Allow it to boil before reducing it to simmer. This should take about 12 minutes or until the chicken is cooked all the way to the center.

6.   Add salt & pepper to taste

Nutrition Facts: contains 196 calories, 10.4g fat, 1.8g fiber, 5.8g carbohydrates, and 26.4g protein

Another Low Carb Keto Chicken Soup

Cooking Time: 30 minutes

Servings: 4 servings

Ingredient List:

- 1 1/4 small yellow onion finely diced
- 2 medium carrots peeled and chopped
- 1 small leek chopped
- 3 medium stalks celery chopped
- 1.5 liters chicken stock
- 1 cup chopped kale
- 1/4 tsp black pepper or to taste
- 1 tbsp butter or extra virgin olive oil
- 1 tbsp thyme leaves chopped
- 300 g cooked chicken

- 2 bay leaves
- 8 g fresh parsley
- 1 garlic clove minced
- Salt to taste
- Squeeze of lemon juice (for serving)
- 1 tbsp olive oil (for serving)
- 1 tsp fresh parsley (for serving)

Instructions:

1. Grab a soup pot and put 1 tablespoon of butter or olive oil. Cook it over medium heat and sauté the onion, celery, leek, carrots, and thyme in the pan. Wait until they start to soften.

2. Put in the stock and bay leaves. Season and raise the heat so that the soup will start to boil.

3. Reduce the heat to a simmer and allow it to cook for 15 minutes or so.

4. Add in the chicken.

5. Optional: remove half of the mixture and pulse it for a few seconds using a stick blender. This is a great way to thicken the soup and promote flavor. Put the soup back afterwards. However, if you don't have a stick blender, you can skip this step entirely.

6. Mix the olive oil with lemon juice and put it in the soup. Place the fresh parsley and season the soup according to your taste.

Nutrition Facts: 286kcalories, 7.6g net carbohydrates, 10.2g carbohydrates, 29g protein, 2.7g fiber, and 395mg sodium

Keto Low Carb Vegetable Soup Recipe

Cooking Time: 35 minutes

Servings: 12 servings

Ingredient List:

- 2 tbsp olive oil
- 1 tbsp Italian seasoning
- 2 cups Green beans trimmed, cut into 1-inch pieces
- 8 cups chicken broth
- 1 large onion, diced
- 2 large Bell peppers diced
- 4 cloves Garlic minced
- 1 medium head Cauliflower cut into 1-inch florets
- 2 14.5-oz cans diced tomatoes
- Salt and pepper to taste

Instructions:

1. Heat olive oil over medium heat using a pot.
2. Put in the bell pepper and onions. Cook for 10 minutes or until the onions become browned.
3. Put in the garlic and cook until fragrant.

4.   Place the 8 cups of chicken broth.

5.   Add the green beans, cauliflower, broth, diced tomatoes, and Italian seasoning. Add salt and pepper to taste

6.   Increase the heat and have the soup boiling before reducing it to a simmer and putting a lid on top. The soup is ready when the green beans are already soft and ready for consumption.

7.   Enjoy!

Nutrition Facts: contains 79kcalories, 2g fat, 2g protein, 11g total carbohydrates, 3g fiber, and 5g sugar

Egg Drop Soup

Cooking Time: 20 minutes

Servings: 6 servings

Ingredient List:

- 4 large eggs
- 2 quarts chicken or vegetable stock
- 1 tbsp grated turmeric
- 1 tbsp grated ginger
- 6 tbsp extra virgin olive oil
- 2 tbsp coconut aminos
- 2 tbsp freshly chopped cilantro

- 1 tsp salt or to taste
- 2 cloves garlic, minced
- 2 cups sliced brown mushrooms
- 4 cups chopped Swiss chard/spinach
- 1 small chili pepper, sliced
- 2 medium spring onions, sliced
- freshly ground black pepper to taste

Instructions:

1.   Put the chicken stock in a large pot. Apply medium heat until it starts to simmer

2.   Put the turmeric, ginger, chili pepper, mushroom, coconut aminos, and char stalks into the pot. Allow it to simmer for 5 more minutes.

3.   Include the sliced chard leaves and allow it to cook for another minute

4.   In a separate bowl, whisk the eggs and then pour them carefully into the soup. Stir constantly until the egg is cooked

5.   Add the chopped cilantro and spring onions to the pot.

6.   Add salt and pepper to taste.

7.   Serve with a drizzle of extra virgin olive oil. You can store this for five days in an airtight container in the fridge.

Nutrition Facts: 255kcalories, 10.8g protein, 2.9g net carbohydrates, and 22.4g fat

Instant Pot Chili Verde

Cooking Time: 40 minutes

Servings: 4 servings

Ingredient List:

- 2 lbs boneless skinless chicken thighs
- 12 oz tomatillos, husked and quartered
- 8 oz poblano peppers stemmed, seeded, and chopped
- 4 oz jalapeño peppers stemmed, seeded, and chopped
- 4 oz onions chopped
- 1/4 cup water
- 1 1/2 tsp salt
- 2 tsp ground cumin
- 5 cloves garlic
- ¼ oz chopped cilantro leaves (for finishing)
- 1 tbsp fresh lime juice (for finishing)

Instructions:

1. Put the poblanos, jalapenos, onions, and tomatillos in a pressure cooker. Add the water and sprinkle the cumin, salt, and garlic on top.

2.   Put the chicken inside and seal the lid.

3.   Turn the pressure on high for 15 minutes.

4.   Release the pressure and uncover the lid. Put the chicken on a cutting board and cut it into small pieces. Set it aside.

5.   Add cilantro and lime juice to the pressure cooker.

6.   Choose the sauté mode on the pressure cooker.

7.   Put the chicken back to the mixture and boil for the next 10 minutes to cause the chicken sauce to thicken. Stir it occasionally.

8.   Serve and garnish with more cilantro if you want.

Nutrition Facts: 310 calories, 15g total fat, 10g total carbohydrates, 37g protein

Keto Salad Recipes

Keto Cobb Salad

Cooking Time: 5 minutes

Servings: 1 serving

Ingredient List:

- 4 cherry tomatoes, diced
- 1 avocado, sliced

- 1 hardboiled egg, sliced
- 2 oz. chicken breast, shredded
- 1 oz. feta cheese, crumbled
- ¼ cup cooked bacon, crumbled
- 2 cups mixed green salad

Instructions:

1. Mix the green salad in a large bowl. Add the chicken breast, feta cheese, and the crumbled bacon.
2. Put the tomatoes, avocado, egg, chicken, bacon, and feta cheese on top of the greens.
3. Enjoy! You can also try adding some ranch dressing but be aware that this adds to the total fat and calorie content of your salad.

Nutrition Facts: contains 412 calories, 23.6g of fat, 264.3mg of cholesterol, 6g of fiber, and 38.4g of protein.

5 Ingredient Keto Salad

Cooking Time: 10 to 15 minutes

Servings: 2 servings

Ingredient List:

- 2 boneless chicken breasts with skin
- 1 large avocado, sliced

- 3 slices of bacon
- 4 cups mixed leafy greens of choice
- 2 tbsp. dairy-free ranch dressing
- Salt and pepper to taste
- Duck fat for greasing

Instructions:

1. Start by preheating the oven to 200 degrees Celsius or 400 degrees Fahrenheit.
2. Season the chicken with salt and pepper. Grab a skillet and grease it with duck fat before cooking the chicken on the hot pan.
3. Keep the heat on high until you get a golden brown skin surface. This should take around 5 minutes per side.
4. Once done, you can cook the chicken in the oven for 10 to 15 minutes. You can also put the bacon in with the chicken to save on the cooking time. You can also fry it in a pan, depending your personal preferences.
5. After cooking, let the chicken rest for a few minutes.
6. Slice the avocado and the cooked chicken.
7. Start assembling your salad, adding together the leafy greens, crispy bacon, sliced chicken, and avocado.
8. Use 2 tablespoons of ranch dressing. Mix together until all ingredients are thoroughly coated. Enjoy!

Nutrition Facts: 3.1g carbs, 38.7g protein, 43.8g fat, and 581 kcalories

Vegetarian Keto Cobb

Cooking Time:

Servings: 3 servings

Ingredient List:

- 3 large hard boiled eggs, sliced
- 4 ounces cheddar cheese, cubed
- 2 tbsp. sour cream
- 2 tbsp. mayonnaise
- ½ tsp. garlic powder
- ½ tsp. onion powder
- 1 tsp. dried parsley
- 1 tbsp. milk
- 1 tbsp. Dijon mustard
- 3 cups romaine lettuce, torn
- 1 cup cucumber, diced
- ½ cup cherry tomatoes, halved

Instructions:

1. The dressing is a combination of the source cream, mayonnaise, and dried herbs. Mix them well together until full combined.

2. Add one tablespoon of milk into the mix until you get the thickness you want.

3. Layer in the salad, adding all the ingredients that's not part of the dressing recipe. Put the mustard on the center of the salad.

4. Drizzle with your dressing and enjoy! Each serving should have just 2 tablespoons of dressing to meet the nutritional information given below.

Nutrition Facts: 330 calories, 26.32g fat, 16.82g protein, and 4.83g net carbohydrates

Keto Chicken Salad w/ Avocado

Cooking Time: 20 minutes

Servings: 2 servings

Ingredient List:

- 2 pcs. of boneless chicken thigh fillets
- 2 tbsp. olive oil
- ¼ cup water
- 1 tsp. salt
- 1 tsp. sweet chili powder

- 1 tsp. dried thyme
- ½ tsp. ground black pepper
- 4 cloves garlic
- Handful of cherry tomatoes (salad)
- 2 cups arugula (salad)
- 1 cup purslane leaves (salad)
- ½ cup fresh dill (salad)
- 1 tbsp. olives (salad)
- 1 tsp. sesame seeds (salad)
- 1 tsp. nigella seeds (salad)
- ½ tbsp. olive oil (salad)
- 2 tbsp. avocado dressing (salad)
- 1 avocado, sliced (salad)
- Basil leaves (salad)

Instructions:

1. Pour ¼ cup of water on a skillet and cook the chicken fillets over medium heat, keeping the lid covered until the water drains completely.

2. Drizzle 2 tbsp. of olive oil on the chicken. Add some garlic cloves and then season it with salt and pepper. Add some thyme and sweet chili powder. Cook them again until golden, making sure you flip the chicken every now and again to even out the sides.

3. Put all the salad ingredients in a bowl. Put in some nigella seeds and sesame seeds with some olive oil and avocado dressing. Mix and enjoy!

Nutrition Facts: contains 1093 calories, 17g of sugar, 81g of fat, 68g protein, and 34g of carbohydrates.

Keto Chicken Salad

Cooking Time: 20 to 25 minutes

Servings: 4 servings

Ingredient List:

- 2 cups cooked chicken, shredded
- 2 boiled eggs, chopped
- ¼ cup pecans, chopped
- ¼ cup dill pickles, chopped
- ½ cup mayonnaise
- ¼ cup minced yellow onion
- 1 tsp. yellow mustard
- 1 tsp. white distilled vinegar
- 1 tsp. fresh dill
- Salt and pepper to taste

Instructions:

1. Except for the chicken, add everything together in a mixing bowl and stir together until thoroughly combined.
2. Add the chicken and stir well, making sure that all of the chicken are well coated.
3. Add salt and pepper to taste.
4. Chill in the fridge for one hour before serving. You can keep it stored in the fridge for 3 to 5 days.

Nutrition Facts: Each serving contains 394 calories, 33g saturated fat, 6g trans fat, 25g cholesterol, 3g carbohydrates, 1g sugar, and 21g protein.

Tuna Fish Salad – Quick and Easy!

Cooking Time: 10 minutes maximum

Servings: 1 serving

Ingredient List:

- 10 kalamata olives, pitted
- 1 small zucchini sliced lengthwise
- ½ diced avocado
- 2 cups of mixed greens
- 1 large diced tomato
- 1 sliced green onion
- 1 can chunk light tuna in water, drained

- ¼ cup fresh parsley, chopped
- ½ cup fresh mint, chopped
- 1 tbsp. extra virgin olive oil
- 1 tbsp. balsamic vinegar
- ¼ tsp. fine sea salt
- ¾ tsp. black pepper, cracked

Instructions:

1. Grill the zucchini slices on both sides for a few minutes or as desired. Once cooked, cut it into bite-size pieces.

2. Grab a large bowl and just put all the ingredients together in the container, mixing them together until the liquid ingredients are evenly distributed.

3. Serve while still fresh. This salad would taste best if eaten immediately so try not to have any leftovers.

Nutrition Facts: contains 563 calories, 30.9g total fat, 37.5g carbohydrates, 15.7g dietary fiber, and 41.8g protein.

Chapter 10: 30-Day Ketogenic Diet Meal Plan

Okay, so you we're given recipes above to help start your journey towards a Keto-friendly diet. I understand however that many of those recipes are a bit more complicated than most – especially if you're a complete beginner. Chances are you're having a hard time with the groceries and the unknown food items that are suddenly included in your grocery list.

While you're strongly encouraged to do some shopping and try out many of the recipes I gave above, I understand how this healthier lifestyle is a bit new to you. This is why in this Chapter, I'm introducing a 30-day diet plan that would be perfect if you're brand new to the lifestyle. The goal of this 30-day diet is to help you blend easily into the Ketogenic Diet without breaking the bank. Many of these recipes will have 8 or less ingredients and should take less than 30 minutes to make.

Preparations: What to Do

Week 1 is the start of the Ketogenic Diet, but that doesn't mean that you start preparing on that same week. Ideally, the preparation process begins a day before the first day of the diet. Why? Well, before the first day, I want you to have everything you need easily within reach.

Step 1: Take a good look at your fridge and figure out what food products do not go with your new Keto-friendly lifestyle. I want you to get rid of those items without throwing them in trash. Maybe donate them to the nearest charity store?

Step 2: Figure out what you want to eat for breakfast, lunch, and dinner on your first week of the Ketogenic Diet. For this, I want you to refer to the chapter on recipes for the simplest and easiest ones to make. If you don't cook often or prefer to make your own dishes, then here's a rough guideline of what you should and should not eat.

Eat: meat including fish, eggs, beef, lamb and poultry; high-fat dairy like cheese, butter, and cream; low-carb vegetables like spinach, broccoli, and kale; avocado and berries; coconut oil, high-fat salad dressing, and substitute sweeteners. This has been explained thoroughly in a previous Chapter and should give you a good jump off point.

In contrast, avoid eating the following: all types of grains, fruits, potato, yams, and sugar like honey and maple syrup.

Step 4: Write down your meals for the entire week. Grab a notebook or any other note-taking tool you have and start planning what you will eat for the next 7 days. While you're perfectly free to choose any day of the week for this, I strongly encourage that you choose a non-busy day. Perhaps the weekend to help you better works in the meals to your plan. Starting on a relaxing day will make it easier for you when changing something important in your lifestyle.

Step 5: Go to the grocery store and start buying what you need based on the meals you've decided to prepare. I want you to understand that you don't have to be overly complicated on this. Even egg fried on butter complies with the Ketogenic Diet so if you're not big on cooking – there's nothing wrong with that!

Step 6: You will basically be repeating all the steps given here on a weekly basis. While you're perfectly welcome to formulate a 30-day meal plan for yourself, it's usually a better idea to take it one week at a time. This will help you get used to the idea and make each week feel easier than the last. Plus, you can make adjustments your routine depending on how the last week turned out.

Week 1: What to Expect

During the first week of your 30-day diet, expect to experience many of the signs of Ketogenic Flu as discussed in a previous Chapter. So you're likely going to feel tired some days and energetic on other days. You'll have headaches, feel thirsty, have days of lightheadedness days, and days when you feel like you can conquer the world.

If you've enjoy a carbohydrate rich diet before jumping into the Ketogenic Diet, then chances are you'll also have some cravings throughout the first few days of the diet. What do you do? You power through it of course! The first 7 days are the toughest so these are actually the days when you want to establish a solid meal plan. Precision is important from your breakfast, lunch, dinner, and snacks.

Why is that? This is because I want you to remove the possibility of bargaining. Your first 7 days in the diet will be tough and you're probably going to tell yourself "I don't have to quit carbohydrates completely – I can just eat 2 Keto-friendly meals and 1 carbohydrate-rich one and still be on the Ketogenic Diet.

I don't want you going through this kind of self-bargaining process because you'll only be fooling yourself. Having a set meal plan during the first 7 days will remove the possibility of you talking yourself out of the situation.

So what happens now? Here, our goal is to keep things simple and leftover friendly. This is important since your first week of dieting shouldn't be so difficult. One of the top reasons why people quit their diet is because it's too hard to follow so we'll try to make sure this isn't an ordeal for you.

So let's do this:

Breakfast Suggestion: Bacon and Eggs

Cooking Time: 5 to 10 minutes

Servings: 4 servings

Ingredient List

- 8 eggs, medium sized
- 5 oz. sliced bacon
- Fresh parsley optional
- Cherry tomatoes optional

Instructions:

- Fry the bacon on medium heat using keto-approved oil and put it aside when crispy.
- Using the same pan, fry the eggs in the remaining bacon grease and oil.
- When the eggs are just about cooked, cut up the tomatoes and put them in with the eggs.
- Remove the eggs from the pan and put parsley on top as wished. Used salt and pepper to taste.

Nutrition Facts:

- 1 gram carbohydrates
- 22 grams fat
- 15 grams protein
- 0 grams fiber
- 272 kcal

Note: We're starting breakfast quick and easy with ingredients that you probably already have. Note though, this makes 4 servings so if you're only eating for yourself, try reducing the ingredients significantly.

Breakfast Suggestion: Low Carb Oatmeal

Cooking Time: 20 minutes

Servings: 1 serving

Ingredient List:

- 1 cup of unsweetened almond milk
- 1/2 cup of hemp hearts
- 1 tsp of flax meal
- 1 tsp of chia seeds
- 1 tsp of coconut flakes
- 1 tsp of cinnamon
- 1 scoop of vanilla MCT oil powder

Instructions:

1. Combine all the ingredients in a large sauce pot. Stir thoroughly.
2. Bring it to a simmer until it gets thick enough to your liking.
3. Garnish with berries and enjoy!

Nutrition Facts: contains 44 grams of fat, 584 calories, 16g fiber, 31g protein, and 17g carbohydrates

Lunch Suggestion: Cauliflower Mac and Cheese

Cooking Time: 30 minutes

Servings: 3 servings

Ingredient List:

- 1 tsp salt
- 1/2 tsp black pepper
- 1 1/4 tsp paprika
- 8 oz heavy cream
- 4 oz sharp cheddar, shredded
- 4 oz fontina, shredded
- 2 oz cream cheese
- 1 large head of cauliflower

Instructions:

1. Start by preheating the oven to 375 degrees Fahrenheit. Grab a baking dish and butter the sides while waiting for the desired temperature.
2. Cut the cauliflower into small pieces, about 1 inch each

3. Steam the cauliflower for 5 minutes until it becomes slightly tender. Drain.

4. In a pot, combine the cheese, cream cheese, salt, pepper, heavy cream, and paprika.

5. Add cauliflower to the cheese mixture. Toss it around to coat everything

6. Pour into the baking dish and bake for 30 minutes.

Nutrition Facts: each serving contains 393 calories, 33g fat, 10f carbohydrates, 14g protein and 4g fiber

Lunch Suggestion: Bacon, Egg, and Spinach Salad

Cooking Time: 10 to 15 minutes

Servings: 2 servings

Ingredient List:

- 3.5 ounces of cooked bacon, crumbled
- 4 cups of baby spinach
- ½ tsp. of Dijon mustard
- 1 ½ tbsp. of red wine vinegar
- 3 tbsp. of extra virgin olive oil
- Salt and pepper to taste

Instructions:

1. Start by boiling the eggs in the saucepan. At the same time, you can cook the bacon in the stovetop using olive oil as your main medium.
2. Set aside the eggs and bacon after cooking.
3. Grab a bowl and whisk the red wine vinegar, olive oil, and mustard together.
4. Add the bacon, eggs, and spinach in the bowl. Toss and serve

Nutrition Facts: each serving contains 397 calories, 21 grams of protein, 33 grams of fat, 1 gram of fiber, and 7 grams of carbohydrates

Note: If you have some leftovers for breakfast, then feel free to eat that instead of this recipe! Remember, we're trying to keep things simple for you.

Dinner: Keto Tuna Plate

Cooking Time:

Servings: 2 servings

Ingredient List:

- 4 eggs
- 2 oz. baby spinach
- 10 oz. tuna in olive oil

- 1 avocado
- ½ cup mayonnaise
- Salt and pepper to taste
- ¼ lemon (optional)

Instructions:

1. Start by boiling the eggs for 4 to 8 minutes, depending on whether you like them soft boiled or hard boiled. Set aside to cool without removing the shell just yet.
2. Put together the spinach and tuna in one place. Put some mayonnaise on the side and if you want lemon, put a wedge on the edge of the plate.
3. Remove the eggshell and add it onto the plate.
4. Add some salt and pepper to taste

Nutrition Facts: each serving contains 3g of net carbohydrates, 7g of fiber, 931 kcalories, 76g of fat, and 52g of protein.

Week 2: What to Expect

You'll notice that there are no dessert recipes for Week 1 – and that's because we're trying to keep the sugar count low. Dessert is OK for the 3rd and 4th week, but unfortunately, the first 2 weeks would be dessert-free. Hence, this week's recipes will be just as simple. Fortunately, you can still snack in between meals if you want.

I really hope you stuck to your dietary routine during the first week. You should be proud of yourself if you stuck to the diet despite the occurrence of the Keto Flu symptoms. You're probably wondering: will it still be present during the second week?

The answer really depends on your personal situation. If you have a lot of weight to lose or if you've been on a carbohydrate-rich diet for years, then the Keto Flu can extend as far as the second week. Again: power through it!

Other things you might expect during the second week are constipation. Increase your water and fiber intake during these days. On the upside, you'll experience better sleep and on some days, you'll enjoy a mental clarity unlike any other. Of course, there will be days of frustration and cravings – but I want you to power through it still! Eat keto-friendly snacks like nuts and avocado to help stave off the cravings. The good news is that you won't be hungry as fat keeps you feeling full for longer periods of time. Cravings however are another matter entirely, but you got this far and you can go further still.

Breakfast Suggestion: Keto Coffee

Cooking Time: 2 minutes

Servings: 16 ounces

Ingredient List:

- 2 cups of hot coffee, freshly brewed
- 2 tbsp grass fed butter
- 1 scoop of Perfect Keto MCT powder
- 1 tsp Ceylon cinnamon

Instructions:

1. Combine all ingredients in a blender
2. Use a frother and blend the mix for 30 seconds or until you get that beautiful frothy consistency.
3. Serve and enjoy!

Nutrition Facts: 280 calories, 31g fat, carbohydrates 2.8g, protein 1g, and 2.2g fiber.

Breakfast Suggestion: Keto Pancakes

Cooking Time: 10 to 15 minutes

Servings: 4 servings

Ingredient List:

- 4 eggs

- 7 oz. of cottage cheese
- 2 oz. butter for cooking
- 1 tbsp. ground psyllium husk powder
- 2 oz. fresh raspberries or blueberries or strawberries
- butter as topping

Instructions:

1. Start by combining the cottage cheese, eggs, and psyllium husk and mixing th7em together. Leave it there for around 5 to 10 minutes to thicken up.
2. Melt the butter in a non-stick skillet using medium heat. Carefully fry the pancake batter, keeping each pancake small so you'd be able to flip them easily.
3. Serve with berries and butter on top. Some people like to use whipped cream as topping and this is also OK as long as you opt for a low-sugar option.

Nutrition Facts: 4 grams of carbohydrates per serving, 3 grams of fiber, 39 grams of fat, 13 grams of protein, and 424 kcalories

Lunch Suggestion: Keto Caesar Salad

Cooking Time: 15 to 20 minutes

Servings: 4 servings

Ingredient List:

- ¾ lb. chicken breasts
- 1 tbsp. olive oil
- 3 oz. bacon
- 7 oz. romaine lettuce, chopped
- 1 oz. parmesan cheese, grated
- Salt and pepper to taste
- ½ cup mayonnaise (for dressing)
- 1 tbsp. Dijon mustard (for dressing)
- ½ lemon zest and juice (for dressing)
- ½ oz. parmesan cheese, grated (for dressing)
- 2 tbsp. anchovies, finely chopped (for dressing)
- 1 garlic clove (for dressing)
- Salt and pepper to taste (for dressing)

Instructions:

1. Preheat the oven to 350 degrees Fahrenheit
2. Mix all the ingredients for the dressing and whisk them into a fine and smooth blend. Set it aside in the fridge.
3. Grab the chicken and season it with salt, pepper, and olive oil. Bake for 20 minutes or until you get the crispiness that you want. Remove and slice according to your personal preferences.
4. Fry the bacon until crispy.

5. Take the chopped lettuce and put it on the plate. Top with chicken and bacon, layering it on the surface for as much as you want.

6. Take the dressing out of the fridge and finish it all off with a small dollop on the side. Grate some parmesan cheese on top and enjoy!

Nutrition Facts: contains 1019 kcalories, 51g protein, 87g fat, and 3g fiber.

Dinner Suggestion: Keto Chicken Burges with Tomato

Cooking Time: 30 minutes

Servings: 4 servings

Ingredient List:

- 1 egg
- 2 oz. butter for frying (for patties)
- 1 ½ lbs. ground chicken (for patties)
- 1 tsp. ground sea salt (for patties)
- ½ yellow onion, grated (for patties)
- ½ tsp. ground black pepper (for patties)
- 1 tsp. dried thyme (for patties)
- 1 ½ lbs. green cabbage

- 3 oz. butter
- 1 tsp. salt
- ½ tsp. ground black pepper
- 4 oz. butter (sauce)
- 1 tbsp. tomato paste (sauce)
- Salt and pepper to taste (sauce)

Instructions:

1. Start by preheating the oven to 220 degrees Fahrenheit
2. Combine all patty ingredients and whisk thoroughly until you achieve a smooth concoction.
3. Shape and fry the patties in butter until cooked. Set them aside. Ideally, you should keep them in the oven so they'll remain warm.
4. Shred the cabbage and fry them on the same skillet where you fried the chicken patties. Season with salt and pepper.
5. Next, you'll be making the tomato butter. Combine all the ingredients for the sauce and whisk them with a handheld mixer.
6. Take the chicken patties back and serve on a plate. The friend cabbage and the tomato butter will be your side dishes and dips. Enjoy!

Nutrition Facts: contains 771 kcalories, 8g of carbohydrates, 5g fiber, 67g fat, and 34g protein.

Week 3: What to Expect

Congratulations for reaching the third week! Around the third week of your diet, you're probably already struggling a little with this whole thing. If you're using Keto Strips, then the reading should wind down by the end of the third week. This means that you'll be positive for Ketosis during the first and 2nd week, but this might not longer be positive on the 3rd week.

For the 3rd week – we're going to do a slight change on your diet. Instead of cooking your breakfast, you'll be drinking your breakfast. Why are we doing this? Well, the third week is the introduction of a very slight fast. Slightly depriving your body of food during the 3rd week can help speed up the fat burning process of the body.

Of course, I want to stress out that the fast is only a good idea if you're actually trying to lose weight. If you're only doing this to keep your health up – then fasting during the 3rd week is NOT advisable. Instead, I want you to take a good look at the recipes already mentioned in the previous Chapter and try those out. Or maybe try out some of the breakfasts you made in the first and second weeks.

Breakfast Suggestion: Strawberry Avocado Keto Smoothie

Cooking Time: 2 minutes

Servings: 1 serving

Ingredient List:

- 1 lb. frozen strawberries
- 1 large avocado
- 1 ½ cup unsweetened almond milk
- ¼ cup erythritol or any other sweetener of your choice

Instructions:

- Puree all the ingredients in a blender. Add with ice and enjoy.

*Nutrition Facts:*106 kcalories

Lunch Suggestion: Keto Cheeseburger

Cooking Time: 15 to 20 minutes

Servings: 4 servings

Ingredient List:

- 2 tomatoes (salsa)

- 2 scallions (salsa)
- 1 avocado (salsa)
- Salt (salsa)
- Fresh cilantro to taste (salsa)
- 1 tbsp. olive oil (salsa)
- 1 ½ lbs. ground beef (burger)
- 7 oz. shredded cheese – divided (burger)
- 2 tsp. onion powder (burger)
- 2 tsp. garlic powder (burger)
- 2 tsp. paprika powder (burger)
- 2 tbsp. fresh oregano, chopped (burger)
- 2 oz. butter for frying (burger)
- 5 oz. lettuce
- ¾ cup mayonnaise
- 4 tbsp. Dijon mustard
- 5 oz. crumbled cooked bacon
- 4 tbsp. pickled jalapenos, chopped
- 2 ½ dill pickles, sliced

Instructions:

1. Start by chopping up all the ingredients meant for the salsa. Add them together in a bowl and set aside.

2. Now focus on the meat. Mix all the seasoning and half of the cheese into a bowl. Mix your raw burger meat thoroughly to distribute the flavor evenly.

3. Divide the meat into 4 patties, forming them into even circles for frying.

4. Once cooked, sprinkle the remaining cheese on top of the patty.

5. Serve with the lettuce, bacon, mayonnaise, jalapeños, mustar, and dill pickle. Make sure to choose your bread properly because bread is packed with carbohydrates. You can try following any of the bread recipes provided in this book or you can purchase a keto-friendly bread option. You can also choose not to have any bread with your patty.

Nutrition Facts: per serving you get 8g of net carbohydrates, 104g fat, 53g protein, 6g fiber, and 1194 kcalories

Dinner Suggestion: Chicken Drumsticks

Cooking Time: 30 minutes to 1 hour

Servings: 1 serving

Ingredient List:

- ½ tbsp. light olive oil
- ½ tbsp. lime juice
- ½ tsp. salt
- 1/8 tsp. cayenne pepper
- ¼ tbsp. smoked paprika powder

- ¼ tbsp. garlic powder
- ¾ lb. chicken drumsticks

Instructions:

1. Start by preheating the oven to 400 degrees Fahrenheit
2. Grab a large bowl and whisk together all the ingredients for the chicken. Once done, marinade the chicken thighs overnight until the juice really seeps into the chicken. Make sure the chicken is completely coated by the liquid.
3. Once done with the chicken, put the drumsticks on a wire rack and bake for 30 minutes. Remove and enjoy!

Nutrition Facts: Includes 11g of net carbohydrates, 4g of fiber, 77g fat, 64g protein, and 1016 kcalories

Note: The beauty of this recipe is that you can keep the uncooked chicken in the fridge for long periods of time. Every time you want dinner, you can take them out of the fridge and pop them in the oven for a quick meal.

Week 4: What to Expect

You're now at the fourth week of your 30-day Ketogenic Meal Plan! I'm really proud of how far you've gone and I want you to know that even if you stumbled along the way, you can still push forward with the Ketogenic Diet.

By the fourth week, your health status should be more good than bad. The signs of the Keto Flu should have subsided so that you're only enjoying the positive effects of the diet.

Breakfast: Cauliflower Hash Browns

Cooking Time: 15 minutes

Servings: 4 servings

Ingredient List:

- 1 lb. cauliflower
- 3 eggs
- 1 tsp. salt
- 2 pinches pepper
- ½ yellow onion, grated
- 4 oz. butter for frying

Instructions:

1. Start by grating the cauliflower or putting it in food processors until you get a rice-like texture.

2. Put the grated cauliflower in a bowl and add all the other ingredients except for the butter, of course. Whisk them all together until you get a nice mixture.

3. Fry the cauliflower the butter. Keep the heat on low to make sure the cauliflower cooks thoroughly without any burnt edges. This should take about 3 to 4 inches per side.

Nutrition Facts: contains 282 kcalories, 5g of carbohydrates, 3g of fiber, 26g of fat, and 7g protein.

Lunch: Low Carb Bakes Eggs

Cooking Time: 5 to 10 minutes

Servings: 1 serving

Ingredient List:

- 3 oz. ground beef
- 2 eggs
- 2 oz. shredded cheese

Instructions:

1. Start by preheating the oven to 400 degrees Fahrenheit

2. Place the ground beef in a baking dish. Press it into the baking dish and create two holes with a spoon. It

should be large enough that you can crack the eggs into the hole.

3. Once cracked, sprinkle some of the cheese on top.
4. Bake the whole thing in the oven for 15 minutes
5. Let it cool before serving. Enjoy!

Nutrition Facts: 2g net carbohydrates, 35g fat, 41g protein, and 498 k calories

Dinner: Strawberry and Spinach Salad

Cooking Time: 10 minutes

Servings: 4 servings

Ingredient List:

- 4 cups cut spinach
- 2 cups sliced strawberries
- ½ cup goat cheese, crumbled
- ¼ cup almonds
- ½ cup mayonnaise (for dressing)
- 1 tbsp. olive oil (for dressing)
- 1 tbsp. white vinegar (for dressing)
- 1 tbsp. poppy seeds (for dressing)
- 2 tbsp. sweetener, hone or maple (for dressing)
- ¼ tsp. sea salt

Instructions:

1. Just add the entire salad ingredients together in one bowl.
2. In a separate bowl, whisk together the dressing ingredients until properly combined. You can thin it out with some water or more oil if you want. Adjust seasoning to taste.
3. Drizzle on your salad and enjoy

Nutrition Facts: contains about 247k calories, 23g fat, 5g carbohydrates, 2g fiber, and just 2g sugar.

Fast Way of life

As much as it pains me to put this in here, I have to consider the likelihood that not everyone has the luxury of time. You may have a demanding career or schedule that makes it difficult for you to prepare your meals every single time. The good news is that there are recipes you can prepare by bulk. For example, the chicken broth recipes can be made in large quantities and just reheated for a meal.

However, what if even that becomes difficult to do? While I strongly DISCOURAGE resorting to fast food or restaurant meals as this would make it difficult to monitor what you eat, I have to consider that there will be days when you have no choice. If or when this happens, here are food items you can order:

- Bunless Burgers – you can order the burgers and just don't eat the buns to significantly lower the carbohydrate content of the food. The good news is that you can do this with practically any burger product, whether it's being served by McDonalds, Burger King or Wendy's. McDonalds also has a nutrition calculator which should help you better choose what food to order when you're out. Their Artisan Grilled Chicken Sandwich without the bun and ketchup only has 2 grams worth of carbohydrates and Wendy's version of the same sandwich also has the same 2g carb count. The Whopper Jr. with no buns and plainly made has ZERO calories.

- Salads – not all salads are created equal. The rule is that you want to avoid the sweet dressings on your salad – no matter how packed it is with fresh greens. Skip the fruits as well or stick to berries instead of the sugary fruit treats. The Chipotle Salad Bowl with steak, romaine cheese, and sour cream has only 7 grams of carbohydrates, 30 grams of protein and 405 calories. Arby's Roast Turkey Farmhouse Salad with buttermilk rank dressing only contains 10 grams of carbohydrates, 22 grams of protein, 35 grams of fat, and 440 calories.

- Burrito Bowls – yes, you can still enjoy some burrito! The Taco Bell Cantina PowerSteak Bowl w/ extra guacamole without the rice & beans only has 8 grams of carbohydrates, 23 grams of fat, 310 calories, and 20 grams of protein. Chipotle's Steak Burrito with the salsa, sour cream, lettuce, and cheese only has 6 grams of carbohydrates while their Chicken Burrito has 10 grams of carbohydrates.

- Egg Breakfasts – Panera Bread's Power Breakfast Bowl of eggs, avocado, tomato, and steak contain all of 5 grams of carbohydrates, 230 calories, and 20 grams of protein. There's also McDonald's Big Breakfast without the hash browns and biscuit which should add up to just 2 grams of carbohydrates, 29 grams of fat, and 19 grams of protein.

Conclusion

Congratulations for making it this far! By now, I trust you already have a good understanding of the Ketogenic Diet and how it applies to you as you enjoy your 50s. Obviously, our goal here is to provide a Keto Diet guideline that works for *you*, taking into account your unique situation so that the best and most effective results can be enjoyed.

So what did we cover in this book? We talked about the Ketogenic Diet, how it works, and how to tackle the problems you might encounter because of this brand new diet change. We also talked about the different recipes you can try out for the Ketogenic Diet and of course, the 30-day meal plan to get you started on this new healthy lifestyle choice.

We also talked about how the Ketogenic Diet applies to your unique situation. Unfortunately, at the age of 50 and above, not all food is good food. That's why we had to talk about how to adjust the Ketogenic Diet in such a way that it works with your unique situation. This is important because I want you to stay healthy even while losing weight.

But I think the most important thing I want you to learn from this book is this: it's never too late to make that change! It's never too late to try something new for self-improvement! Don't get set in your ways, especially if your old ways don't do much for your overall health. I want you to know that you have what it takes to be better not just physically, but also mentally and psychologically. Of course, the mere fact that you purchased and read this book is a good start. I know you can do it – all you have to do is take that first important step.

So what should you do next now? I want you to go to the kitchen and take a long good look at the refrigerator. I want you to start evaluating its contents and make a distinction between what's good for you, and which aren't based on the Ketogenic Diet we just discussed. I want you to take that very important first step of deciding on a Keto-friendly breakfast, lunch, and dinner for tomorrow. Choose from any of the recipes mentioned above or choose any method you deem best!

Thank you

Before you go, I just wanted to say thank you for purchasing my book.

You could have picked from dozens of other books on the same topic but you took a chance and chose this one.

So, a HUGE thanks to you for getting this book and for reading all the way to the end.

Now I wanted to ask you for a small favor. **Could you please consider posting a review on the platform? Reviews are one of the easiest ways to support the work of authors.**

This feedback will help me continue to write the type of books that will help you get the results you want. So if you enjoyed it, please let me know.

Resources:

- Steen, J. (2017, March 2). Here's A Simple Explainer On The Ketogenic Diet. Retrieved December 22, 2019, from https://www.huffingtonpost.com.au/2017/03/01/heres-a-simple-explainer-on-the-ketogenic-diet_a_21726260/

- Westman, E. C. (2008, December 19). The effect of a low-carbohydrate, ketogenic diet versus a low-glycemic index diet on glycemic control in type 2 diabetes mellitus. Retrieved December 22, 2019, from https://nutritionandmetabolism.biomedcentral.com/articles/10.1186/1743-7075-5-36

- Campos MD, M. (2019, July 30). Ketogenic diet: Is the ultimate low-carb diet good for you? Retrieved December 22, 2019, from https://www.health.harvard.edu/blog/ketogenic-diet-is-the-ultimate-low-carb-diet-good-for-you-2017072712089

- (Elham Moghaddam, 2006). The Effects of Fat and Protein on Glycemic Responses in Nondiabetic Humans Vary with Waist Circumference, Fasting Plasma Insulin, and Dietary Fiber Intake

- Manninen, A. (2019, December 22). Metabolic Effects of the Very-Low-Carbohydrate Diets: Misunderstood "Villains" of Human Metabolism. Retrieved December 22, 2019, from https://www.ncbi.nlm.nih.gov/pmc/articles/PMC2129159/

- Masood, W. (2019, March 21). Ketogenic Diet - StatPearls - NCBI Bookshelf. Retrieved December 23, 2019, from https://www.ncbi.nlm.nih.gov/books/NBK499830/

- pubmeddev, & Bueno, NB1. (2013). Very-low-carbohydrate ketogenic diet v. low-fat diet for long-term weight loss: a meta-analysis of randomised controlled trials. - PubMed - NCBI. Retrieved December 23, 2019, from https://www.ncbi.nlm.nih.gov/pubmed/23651522

- pubmeddev, & Paoli, A1. (2012). Nutrition and acne: therapeutic potential of ketogenic diets. - PubMed - NCBI. Retrieved December 23, 2019, from https://www.ncbi.nlm.nih.gov/pubmed/22327146

- Allen, B. G. (2019, December 23). Ketogenic diets as an adjuvant cancer therapy: History and potential mechanism. Retrieved December 23, 2019, from https://www.ncbi.nlm.nih.gov/pmc/articles/PMC4215472/

- pubmeddev. (2010). Effects on coronary heart disease of increasing polyunsaturated fat in place of saturated fat: a systematic review and meta-analysis of randomized ... - PubMed - NCBI. Retrieved December 23, 2019, from https://www.ncbi.nlm.nih.gov/pubmed/20351774

- Dashti, H. M. (2004). Long-term effects of a ketogenic diet in obese patients. Retrieved December 23, 2019, from https://www.ncbi.nlm.nih.gov/pmc/articles/PMC2716748/

- Hallböök, T. (2012, July 1). The effects of the ketogenic diet on behavior and cognition. Retrieved December 23, 2019, from https://www.ncbi.nlm.nih.gov/pmc/articles/PMC4112040/

Printed in Great Britain
by Amazon

55734058R00118